Medicine in the Intermountain West

A History of Health Care in Rural Areas of the West

Ward B. Studt, M.D.
Jerold G. Sorensen
Beverly Burge

Foreword by
Bond Bible, Ph.D.

Olympus Publishing Company Salt Lake City, Utah

Development of this publication was supported by Grant No. 5G03 RM000015-08 from the Regional Medical Programs Service. However, its contents are solely the responsibility of the Intermountain Regional Medical Program and are in no way the responsibility of the Regional Medical Programs Service, the Bureau of Health Planning and Resources Development, or the Department of Health, Education, and Welfare.

The Intermountain Regional Medical Association contributed to the funding of this book.

Library of Congress Cataloging in Publication Data

Studt, Ward B 1925-
Medicine in the intermountain West.

Includes index.
1. Medicine — Rocky Mountain region — History. 2. Medicine — Great Basin — History. 3. Rural health services — Rocky Mountain region. 4. Rural health services — Great Basin. 5. Rocky Mountain region — Rural conditions. 6. Great Basin — Rural conditions. I. Sorenson, Jerold G., 1933- joint author. II. Burge, Beverly, 1951- joint author. III. Title.
R152.S87 362.1'0978 76-28520

ISBN 0-913420-66-2

Contents

List of Tables

List of Figures

Foreword

About 56,000,000 people reside in rural America. They are located in all parts of the United States, from the West and the Intermountain West to the Northeast and the South. Some rural residents lack goods and services considered essential to quality living. A basic aspect of quality living is access to good health care.

Rural health care, particularly in the sparsely populated and remote areas, lags behind that of large urban centers. Physician maldistribution continues to be a subject of nationwide interest, particularly the relative deficiency of physicians in rural areas.

The roots of these conditions can be traced to 1900, when parallel threads of technological development created a revolution in agriculture, medicine, and health, with many benefits but also some harmful effects, especially in the delivery of rural health care. The depopulation of the rural countryside started as technology made large-scale farming possible and small-scale farming inefficient by comparison. At the same time, advancing technology in medicine was beginning to require a larger and larger population base to support comprehensive, high-quality health services. Acute deficiencies in rural health manpower were apparent by 1950 as young physicians failed to replace the retiring country doctors.

A significant reversal of the trend toward population outmigration from rural areas occurred during 1970–73 when the total growth rate of nonmetropolitan areas (4.2 percent) exceeded the growth rate of metropolitan centers (2.9 percent). With the energy crisis stimulating the coal industry and with expanded demands for food products, this pattern of rural population growth may continue. The anticipated growth will probably occur in the medium-size county-seat towns, with corresponding need for more health manpower.

Despite the handicaps of rural conditions, individual physicians in solo practice or in a group practice arrangement with other physicians provide adequate, integrated medical care for many people. These doctors often train their own medical assistants and develop a helping relationship with their colleagues in the area. Usually they function with, and have access to, expert specialists and often serve their patients by integrating these widely scattered services. Throughout our nation's history, the individual practitioner has carried on as one of the vanguards of medical care for the American family. *Medicine in the Intermountain West* attests to this fact.

The historical account of medical folkways described, including the use of old home remedies and folk practitioners, still compete with more sophisticated methods of treatment, especially among the low-income rural minorities.

It is certain that many small communities which once had their "own" physician will never again have one of their own. It has become clear that for some sparsely populated rural areas, solutions completely different from the traditional physician in residence must be sought. In some areas, emphasis may be needed on expanded transportation and communication capabilities, use of new allied health professionals, better understanding of individual health practices, and development of emergency care and self-help methods to ensure rural health coverage. Multiple communities in a logical service area will need to plan together to develop health care systems on an area basis so that they can attract appropriate health manpower working in a group to provide home, clinic, and hospital care.

Today, organizing health care systems in sparsely populated areas requires multi-institutional arrangements on a geographical basis. To accomplish this will require courage and foresight on the part of community leaders and health care professionals. Some institutions may have to change their missions or actually close down. Some must be helped to expand. Ambulatory, primary care, and group practice units must be built. Rescue squads must have trained staffs and new equipment to handle acute emergencies until they reach the appropriate hospital. No rural community can handle its problems alone.

Mechanisms need to be developed through which the outreach of health personnel and organizations in high-manpower communities can be extended to communities where manpower is scarce or lacking. Area health education centers might serve as the pattern to be established. This would involve the development of a network of facilities and services through which citizens of low-manpower communities could be referred to appropriate physicians in high-manpower communities on a systematic basis. In all such programs, however, two elements would be central: (1) the location of centers in communities where the social and economic resources are sufficient to sustain a medical center, and (2) the development of medical organizations that would assume responsibility for the medical welfare of citizens in a specified number of communities.

The principal resource of any area is its people, and the ultimate goal of any program is to raise the level of human well-being. Remedial health services are indispensable to the pursuit of that goal. But in the long run, self-maintenance of health and prevention of disease are at least as necessary.

Education for health, then, is a fundamental aspect of community health services and is basic to every health program. Our land grant universities, through their cooperative and university-wide extension services, and other educational institutions must give major emphasis to health education for rural residents directed toward fostering desired changes not only in individual health attitudes and practices, but in use and improvement of community health delivery systems. All of us must recognize that "health does not exist in a vacuum." Health is but one aspect of the "quality of life" which includes all the socioeconomic, ecological, and educational factors which make for a satisfactory living situation. To improve rural health, we must also address the totality of deficiencies in rural living today.

— Bond Bible

Director of the Department of Rural and Community Health, American Medical Association
Secretary of the Council on Rural Health

Preface

Historically, access to good health care has always been a problem in the rural areas of the Intermountain West and, in fact, in the rural United States as a whole. Actually, it made little difference whether one lived near a budding city or in the middle of the desert in the very early days. Medical knowledge was as sparse as the population, and any medical care received was likely to be of questionable value. As the budding cities began to flower, so did the multitude of reasons that brought more physicians and better medical care to these little towns. The rural population remained stagnant or decreased slowly, however, and so did its medical care.

Today the need for improved medical care delivery is considered to be greater in rural areas than in cities. For a variety of reasons studied by numerous commissions and committees throughout the years, rural people do not have the same opportunities for health care as do urban people. Admittedly, rural and urban areas differ widely in their characteristics; but generally speaking, in rural areas the physician shortage is more acute, persons must travel longer distances to obtain health care, emergency health services are more deficient, work-related injury rates are higher, and often a comprehensive approach to health care delivery is not present.

To compound the problem, the Intermountain Region is either mountainous, desert, or semi-desert, and a substantial number of the small communities are many miles apart, a hundred or two hundred miles from the nearest city of twenty thousand to fifty thousand population, and often separated by desert or rugged mountains. Highways are frequently two lanes only, and may traverse mountain passes of seven thousand to ten thousand feet in elevation, where winter driving is hazardous and unpredictable. Regular air transportation exists only between the dozen or so largest cities.

Per capita income of the region is low, with income from manufacturing among the lowest in the nation. The tax base is small, and tax revenues are minimal. Consequently, states in the Intermountain Region are seriously handicapped in trying to improve health care resources by themselves, particularly in nonurban areas.

These facts and much of the information in this book resulted from a study of rural health care began in 1973 by the Intermountain Regional Medical Program. The most astonishing discovery of all was that little material could be found. General information on physician maldistribution was available (as it is for almost all other areas); a few books dealing with specific periods of time included rural references, as did magazine articles (which furnished a few bits and pieces of data). But nowhere was there even an outline about the Intermountain Region's rural health care.

This suggested to us that a published version of the study would be of value. It was felt that the most functional way to present our findings would be in book form. We began gathering information, not fully realizing what a monumental task this really was – that it was a two- or three-year project that would have to be completed in the one year's allotted time. But it was an interesting task and, we feel, a worthwhile one.

Research into old books and articles that had even the vaguest references to medical care explained how rural people coped with their medical problems in the days when a home remedy was not so different from a physician's treatment. We discovered that military men had sat over stone pots to steam away social diseases, that some Mormons had shunned medical treatments and instead had practiced "the laying on of hands." And we found that miners had used whiskey as a cure-all for the diseases they had picked up when they spat on the saloon floors and then slept in the filth they had created.

As the states in the Intermountain Region slowly began to acquire towns and even a few cities, the picture of health care began to change. The automobile was becoming increasingly common and was first seen as transportation for potentially better rural health care. But it was best suited to city streets, not dirt roads – and it actually took more physicians *from* the rural areas than *to* them.

City growth demanded health regulations, some of which spilled over into the rural areas. The Pure Food and Drug Act of 1906 banned foods that were wrongly labeled or that had harmful ingredients. In some ways this protected rural inhabitants, but they still relied heavily on their own products, much more so than urbanites. The Sheppard-Towner Act of 1921 mandated better care for infants and mothers. In Utah, this plan was headquartered in Salt Lake City, but the board of health enlisted the aid of the women's Relief Society of the Church of Jesus Christ of Latter-day Saints (LDS) to help care for the rural areas. The recently established Carnegie Foundation decided to do something about undependable medical education, and the result was the Flexner Report, a document that especially affected medical education in Colorado and helped turn out better qualified physicians for urban and rural areas alike.

Then the Depression hit, and farmers were among those receiving the hardest blow. The government started a program which gave loans to farmers to help them regain sound economic footing, but poor health caused many either to sell some of their government-bought pigs and plows or to decrease their production because they could not work as hard or as often. Realizing that good health care might be the key to success, officials of the Farm Security Administration developed a program of medical cooperatives that gave prepaid and low-cost health care to many farmers in the Intermountain Region. A few private medical cooperatives were also established in rural areas, as farmers sought additional ways to protect their families from hardship.

As the Depression gave way to World War II, and as the war came to an end, people had time to think of such problems as lack of health care, realizing that rural health care was not equal to urban health care. They pressed for projects to upgrade rural health care, and the American Medical Association established a national rural health council. The Sears Foundation set up a plan to attract doctors to rural areas. Medical schools developed programs specifically directed at rural patients and physicians. Individuals crusaded for better rural health too, with the most prominent example in the Intermountain West being Colorado's Dr. Florence Sabin.

Despite the substantial and continuing increase in interest and activity, the problem of rural health care has not been completely resolved. We have attempted to treat this ebb and flow, and we have discussed many rural health care problems, showing how they relate to the Intermountain Region, using statistical material as backup.

The reader should be aware that the statistical information presented in this book is not all for the same year, which for comparative purposes would have been preferred (even though, as one Montana official told us, "rural health statistics don't change that quickly around here"). As a practical matter, obtaining such information would have been virtually impossible, inasmuch as statistical sources were not uniformly available. However, we hope that we have made it clear to our readers when statistical material for different years is used so that they will understand that they are comparing relative situations in the states — not exact situations for the same year.

For ease of comparison, we have separated the counties into those that are rural (100 percent), predominantly rural (50 percent or more), and predominantly urban. According to the Census Bureau's definition of rural, a single community of 2,500 or more population in a county (i.e., one small town, perhaps miles from a city) can cause a county to be classified as urban. Therefore, two sparsely populated states in the Intermountain Region, Nevada and Wyoming, are classified as being basically urban areas (although they have rural characteristics and all of the attendant problems of rural areas throughout the country). In discussing the ages of physicians in Wyoming, for example, we show that many of the more urban areas had physicians with older average ages, which is usually not the case in urban areas. However, in many cases these counties — although technically "urban" — are still very rural.

Two Utah counties, Juab and Grand, are another example of inherently rural areas having been classified as "urban." The total populations in these two counties are 4,500 and 6,600 respectively (rounded to the nearest thousand). They are classified as urban counties, yet 33.3 and 22.7 percent (respectively) of their population are rural. Nephi (Juab County) has a population of 2,699, and the remainder of this slender east-west county is desert. The other towns in Juab County have far less inhabitants than Nephi. A parallel situation exists in Grand County, in Utah's southeast corner, where Moab is the county seat. Moab's population is 4,793, more than two-thirds of the county's total population.

While examining statistics, one must remember that these numbers are averages for the entire state or country. A state in the Intermountain Region can be shown as having a substandard housing rate slightly lower than the national average. Does that mean that this state's housing is probably good? Before deciding what the statistic means, remember that the lowest socioeconomic standards in the rural U.S. today are generally in the southern states and the Appalachia region. Those areas tend to lower the national averages, and by contrast the other regions appear to be high. Also, if the average rural income for a state is low, not all rural areas in that particular state will necessarily be poor. Statistics are not only difficult to interpret sometimes, but they can present other problems. When housing is discussed, for example, it is hard to imagine what "15 percent substandard" really means, unless you are one of those 15 percent. Even then, numbers don't seem to matter. What does matter is that your family is living in unsafe and often unhealthy conditions, and that for a variety of reasons, there often is little you can do about it.

But presenting statistics is one of the few practical ways to give a picture of rural health. It would be much more accurate, and convincing, if we could visit all of our region's rural areas. However, such a trip would be impractical for many of us. Therefore, we hope that, if it is at all possible, we have used these facts and figures to show not only the rural Intermountain West's health situation in numbers, but in terms that really matter – human terms.

The last part of the book examines several recent and successful rural health projects. It is the purpose of this section to show that other rural areas have been able to improve their rural health care situation and to present ideas that have been tried in the Intermountain Region plus others that perhaps, with some adaptation, might be workable in the underserved Intermountain Region. In at least one instance, an avant-garde effort of this type is having considerable success in the Intermountain states, and we have discussed it in some detail.

Conversations with people involved with these projects and other individuals committed to health care of rural people proved interesting. Almost all were extremely kind in giving up time from busy schedules, but several were hesitant about being quoted, for those who have tried the hardest to change the status quo of rural medical delivery have often met with the most criticism. This kept many interesting comments out of the book. Nonetheless, many progressive ideas were expressed by most of these people, plus a small amount of provincialism by others, a "you take care of yours and we'll take care of ours" attitude, which, it has been said, is partly what keeps innovative changes in medicine out of the rural areas.

Despite all of our research and all of the writing, however, this is far from being a total story on rural health in the Intermountain West. Much of the information died with the people who experienced it or, as with information on some government programs, was destroyed. In reality, this is too complex a topic to thoroughly cover in just one year of work. Therefore, we are presenting this book as an overview, not a comprehensive study, for we realize that many rural health programs not mentioned have been tried, and many of the problems and solutions have not been discussed.

We found the story of rural health care in the Intermountain Region to be an interesting one, and we hope that this book will spur even more interest and much more activity in trying to solve the problems.

— *The Authors*

Acknowledgments

The efforts of several people and the words of many went into the final manuscript for this book. The authors would like to thank all of them; yet any list we could devise would inevitably be incomplete.

Tim M. Beaver deserves our appreciation for his many hours of statistical research and for the vast amount of time spent in libraries where he sought any information that had even the most tenuous relationship to health in the Intermountain West.

Bond Bible, Ph.D., director of the American Medical Association's Department of Rural and Community Health and secretary of the Council on Rural Health, was gracious enough to provide considerable material on rural health problems that plague the Intermountain Region, and he also contributed the foreword to this book.

Many others showed immense interest in this project and donated substantial time to our interviewers via telephone calls, in person, and through correspondence: Lillian Allen, D. Ivo Eames, Dr. Fred Humphrey, Dorthea Dolan, Dr. Charles Huff, Dr. and Mrs. Joseph Parker, Pearl Butt, Eldon Billings, Dorothy Lowman, A. J. Redd, Ethel A. Taylor, Dr. Kenneth Castleton, Dr. Paul Crellin, Dr. Edward Gibbs, Dr. H. L. Schiess, and Arvilla Warren.

We also appreciate the help given by the staffs of the University of Utah's Eccles Memorial and Marriott libraries. Without the aid of the Intermountain Regional Medical Association staff – especially secretaries Pam Rogers, Betty Powers, Jeanne Meyer, and Carol Blucher – and the work of the Health Systems Research Institute staff, secretary Kathy Anderson in particular, the manuscript might not have been put into such good, readable form.

Special gratitude is extended to Gary Belch and Merrilee Nielson for their many hours of tedious, yet voluntary, proofreading.

The authors are aware that this book constitutes but a microcosm of the events that were the forerunners of modern-day medicine in the Intermountain West; but we trust that its examples will stimulate other writers to chronicle additional events in the development of medical services. This type of literature is vital if subsequent generations are to benefit from the experiences of those who first brought the art of medicine to western America.

Dedication

To old Doc Parker —

Physician, Soldier,
Raconteur Extraordinaire:

He knew Telluride when the
Ghosts were all alive!

1

Medical Practice – The Dawning

Chickens scattered, squawking their protest, as Dr. William Morse hard-reined his lathered horse, leapt from the saddle amid the swirling dust, and dashed into the two-room log cabin that served as a farmhouse. It had been a hot twenty-mile ride from Cedar City to Parowan in this Utah sun. He had been summoned (as a last resort, he was sure) to David Bulloch's bedside where he found the young man writhing with severe stomach pain. One look at Dave told Morse that he must work swiftly if he were to save the young man's life.

A man of ingenuity, Morse believed in using whatever was available in any given circumstance, and so he bade David's father fetch a live chicken from the yard. The doctor took a sharp knife from his pocket as Bulloch returned. He took the chicken from Bulloch and slit it from its soft underbelly through its breast bone and up to the neck. He whipped the bird open and pressed its still convulsing body onto Dave's bare abdomen. Warm blood trickled down David's sides and onto the quilt. The chicken slowly gave up its protestations.

"Dave," he said, "if it is inflammation of the bowels, I think I can cure you; but if it is mortification, all the doctors in Hades can't save you." To the father he said, "Get me another chicken and keep 'em comin' till I tell you to quit."

As soon as the first chicken's body heat had lessened somewhat, Bulloch handed Dr. Morse another chicken. This procedure was repeated again and again throughout the day and most of the night. By morning the cabin resembled a slaughterhouse and David's body and the bed were saturated with blood, but the pain had subsided. Within a few days the young man was doing his chores as if he'd never experienced a bout with death.

Morse and Bulloch are but two of the many early immigrants to the Intermountain Region, people of courage and determination who headed west with the hope that they would find a better life, or perhaps just find adventure. But newcomers soon found that their aspirations were to be tempered with reality: disease, accidents, death – problems that the pioneers faced alone or in small groups because they were far removed from established cities and all man-made comforts. There were no hospitals and few trained medical men or women. But even if these had existed in the early days of the West, their assistance would have been little more than worthless, for medical facilities were nonexistent and the crude methods such as described above (Doc Morse's chicken poultice) were more provincial than professional. It was truly the time of the Medical Dark Ages; and while the faint glimmering of light was near, most of these immigrants would perish before the dawning of an enlightened medical expertise would find this remote area.

Early People and Practices in the West

Explorers. The first to trek through the American West were the early explorers. From 1804 to 1806, Lewis and Clark crossed the vast Louisiana Purchase twice, and only one man in their party died. Other than sheer luck, this fact can be attributed to President Jefferson's order that both Lewis and Clark receive medical training before they undertook the journey.

Most of the illnesses recorded on these explorations concerned Captain Lewis and the Shoshone Indian woman, Sacajawea, who acted as interpreter and aided the men in finding medicinal herbs. In June 1805, Lewis experienced such pain and fever that he couldn't walk. He ordered one of his men to boil twigs from the chokeberry they found along the trail. This produced a black, bitter tea which Lewis drank every hour, a pint each time. According to his journal, after four doses he was well.

During the trek Sacajawea endured a long, hard labor until a French trader named Jessomme suggested she be given the pulverized rattle of a rattlesnake. Within minutes, she delivered a baby. She also suffered from a tendency toward colds and from intestinal trouble which was worsened by another tendency – she liked to overeat. Lewis treated her with doses of sulfur water, "barks and opium, 'diluted nitre' and boiled buffalo which she ate . . . as heartily as I am willing to permit" (Phillips, 1962).

Traders and Trappers. Fur traders and trappers followed the explorers; their medicine was equally strange and even more crude. The only surgical instrument used (or available) was the knife, and the only anesthetic was whiskey – and plenty of it. The principal medical problems were not diseases, they were gunshot wounds and muscle sprains. If an operation was necessary, the injured person himself performed it, or he was helped by a companion.

Traders adopted sweat baths; typically, covered holes in the earth where the patient would stand for twenty minutes in steam from water poured over heated rocks. Then he would be "immediately plunged twice in cold water and brought back to the hole, where he would resume the vapor bath" (Phillips, 1962). They also used herbs, poultices, and teas, supplementing these faithfully with the ever-present whiskey, and got along as best they could. Health conditions were generally good in those days, for the people who migrated west were mostly young and vigorous and the air and land were pure and fresh.

Frontier Physicians. Periodically, "certified" doctors filtered into the settlements of the West. Dr. John H. Robinson, a volunteer surgeon, traveled through Colorado from 1805 to 1809 with Zebulon Pike. The first doctor to enter the boundaries of present-day Idaho was Dr. Jacob Wyeth. He arrived at Pierre's Hole with the Nathaniel Wyeth exploration party on July 8, 1832; but Dr. Wyeth's twofold problem, dislike for the area and diarrhea, made his stay a short one. Dr. William Stuckley, a naturalist and surgeon, explored Montana with General Isaac I. Stevens in 1853. Reports of that journey reveal that Stuckley spent more time collecting plants then he did in medically treating patients.

The only other trained "doctors" to travel west in the first part of the nineteenth century were missionaries who came to convert the Indians and found themselves taking care of medical problems at the same time. Before he came to St. Mary's Mission in Montana's Bitter Root Valley in 1805, Father Anthony Ravalli of Italy had studied medicine for a time at the University of Padua. He adopted the Indian herbal remedies and then improved upon them by preserving them in alcohol which he distilled from camas roots.

Marcus Whitman, an American physician, pioneer, and missionary, made his way through the Intermountain Region and on to the Oregon Territory three times, in 1835, '36, and '43. While traveling through Wyoming in 1835, he operated on mountaineer Jim Bridger who, as a result of a skirmish with Blackfoot Indians, had been carrying an arrowhead in his back for three years. According to Drury (1973), the Reverend Samuel Parker, who made the trip with Whitman, reported:

> It was a difficult operation because the arrow was hooked at the point by striking a large bone, and a cartilaginous substance had grown around it. The Doctor pursued the operation with great self-possession and perseverance; and his patient manifested equal firmness.

This was perhaps the first operation west of the Rockies performed by an American-trained doctor, and was undertaken eleven years before anesthesia was demonstrated in the United States.

Whitman and his wife Narcissa gave religious training to the Indians and dealt with their medical problems. Traditionally, the Cayuse and the Nez Perce had medicine men called *te-wats*; also by tradition, relatives of the sick were allowed to kill the *te-wat* whose treatment did not result in a cure. This custom put Whitman under constant threat of death.

In 1847, a wagon train brought an epidemic of measles with it. Whitman's medicine kept the white children alive, but the Indian youngsters had no immunity to the disease and many died. The Cayuse believed Whitman to be poisoning their children and in revenge murdered him, his wife, and twelve others.

The Mormons. Meanwhile, the first permanent settlers were making their way to the West. The same year that Whitman was killed, 143 members of the Church of Jesus Christ of Latter-day

Saints (Mormons) arrived in the Salt Lake Valley. The Mormon religion indeed influenced the peoples' attitudes toward medicine and made their health care distinct from other early settlers of the period. The leaders of their church taught them that illnesses were of their own making and could be avoided if they would live the word of God and shun liquor, tobacco, tea and coffee, and other vices. Their prophet, Brigham Young, advocated spiritual healing or the "laying on of hands," a practice explained in his address given in Ogden, Utah, in 1872, when he told how the principle worked (Divett, no date):

> When I lay hands on the sick, I expect the healing power and influence of God to pass through me to the patient and the disease to give way. I do not say that I heal everybody I lay hands on; but many have been healed under my administration. Jesus on one occasion said: "Who has touched me?" A woman had crept up behind Him in the crowd and touched the hem of His garment, and He knew it because the virtue was gone from Him. Do you see the reason and propriety of laying hands on each other? When we are prepared, when we are holy vessels before the Lord, a stream of power from the Almighty can pass through the tabernacle of the administrator to the system of the patient, and the sick are made whole; the headache, fever, or other disease has to give way.

The early Mormons were anti-physician. Brigham Young had told them that instead of calling for a doctor, they should "administer to [the sick] by the laying on of hands and the anointing of oil, giving them mild herbs, and food and medicines that you understand" (Morrell, 1956). Another time, he told them (*Journal of Discourses*, 1873):

> Would you want doctors? Yes, to set bones. We should want a good surgeon for that, or to cut off a limb. But do you want doctors? For not much of anything else, let me tell you.... I will tell you what to do, you ladies, when you find you are going to have an increase, go off into some country where you cannot call for a doctor, and see if you can keep it. I guess you will have it, and I guess it will be all right, too.

Mormons looked down on anyone who did not earn a living by honest toil; doctors were included in this classification. At one time a doctor from Illinois wrote to Brigham Young, volunteering to bring a large group of his neighbors to Utah as converts to

Mormonism. Young told him that if he wanted to earn his bread like an honorable man, he would be welcome, but that there was little need for doctors in Utah.

The general sentiment of the LDS people was well expressed in the *Deseret News* (the official LDS church newspaper) on September 18, 1852 (Alter, 1942):

> Two physicians have removed to one of our most distant settlements and gone to farming; three more have taken to traveling and exploring the country; three have gone to California to dig gold or for some other purpose; and one has gone to distilling, and we are beginning to get some alcohol, which is desirable for gentlemen's shoe blacking, hatter's water proofing, chemical analysis, washing of the bodies of the well to prevent sickness and the sick that they may be made well, when such there be. The physicians who remained have very little practice and will soon have less (we hope).

Midwives. Few people at that time had any knowledge of health care or hygiene; thus the Mormons relied on God, home remedies, and midwives. Common opinion was that a man other than her husband in a woman's bedchamber was an obvious breach of privacy and a humiliating experience for her and her family. The *Deseret News* (September 18, 1852) quoted the Salt Lake Council of Health as saying:

> An adulterous spirit prompts the desire for a doctor instead of a female nurse to wait on [women] when they are sick; and the doctor who delights in nursing women, instead of instructing them to wait on themselves and each other, is possessed of the same spirit.

The demand for midwives increased in the Salt Lake Valley and in other settlements of the Intermountain West. They delivered babies, "laid out" the dead, and cared for the sick. Their home remedies had been handed down through generations of midwifery or had been discovered through trial and error. One Mormon midwife, Patty Session, was renowned for her salve for sores, which contained bark of indigo weed root, boiled down, some beeswax and mutton tallow, and a touch of resin. Paulina Phelps Lyman, who started her medical practice when she was more than sixty years of age, used linseed oil on the blistered face of a little girl who had been playing with a can of gunpowder when it accidently ignited. Mrs. Lyman covered the oil with a mask and then varnished the mask. According to Mrs. Lyman's son William, not a scar was to be seen on the child's face.

Still another Mormon midwife was Ellis Shipp, who taught courses in obstetrics in the late 1880s to women throughout the West and even Mexico and Canada. She also had a "cure" for alcoholism, a mixture of half an ounce of ground quassia steeped in a pint of vinegar. Her prescription was a teaspoonful every time the patient felt a desire for liquor. She claimed that this mixture satisfied the craving for alcoholic beverages and produced a feeling of stimulation and strength. (Quassia is used today in brewing as a substitute for hops.)

Miners and Prospectors. In the 1850s, following the gold strikes in California and Nevada, the Intermountain West was deluged by miners and prospectors, particularly in Montana and Colorado. Miners relied on home cures for most ailments but would seek the advice of doctors who practiced medicine when they, too, were not panning for gold. Last Chance Gulch, later to become Helena, Montana, was one of the more famous mining towns after gold was discovered there in 1864. The town soon had twelve hundred settlers, including twenty men who used the title "doctor." However, since there were no medical licensing laws or medical regulations at that time, anyone who could read a book about medicine, or who perhaps was intrigued by the profession or by the money, was eligible.

Gunshot wounds were common in the not-too-lawful mining camps. Dr. Erasmas D. Leavitt practiced in the Salmon River country of Idaho, and was once called to treat a serious gunshot injury. He not only removed the bullet and fragments of clothing, but parts of the pistol handle as well.

In Montana, Dr. Jerome Glick was summoned to a hideaway to treat Henry Plummer, a bandit leader whose trigger arm had been put out of commission by a sheriff. The bullet had entered the back of Plummer's elbow and passed down the arm, breaking both bones and making his wrist useless. Glick recommended amputation, but Plummer would have nothing to do with that. Two of his men then pulled out their guns and one told Glick: "If Plummer dies, I'll blow your head off!" With this in mind, Glick painstakingly pieced the fractured bones together and was then kept in the cabin until Plummer's recovery was certain. After two months, the bandit leader was well enough so that Glick could leave and the bandits could go back to gunning for the sheriff (Dunlop, 1965).

Accidental injuries were even more common than gunshot wounds in the mining camps. Men fell down mine shafts or were blasted by exploding powder or crushed by falling boulders. Accidents because of drunkenness were frequent, and sometimes even the doctors were under the influence. Seymour Day, who practiced in Red Mountain City, Montana, had a favorite pastime of getting plenty to drink; yet he would never treat a patient while he was inebriated. "Wait until I'm sober," he would say, and then take his own prescribed dosage of three tablespoons of black pepper mixed with whiskey.

But there were also the teetotaling physicians such as Dr. George Kenny of Helena. When some hard-drinking miners demanded that the doctor join in, Kenny grabbed the whiskey bottle and chased them round the room in a vigorous effort to show them just how deadly the effects of alcohol could be (Dunlop, 1965).

Exposure and sudden changes in the weather gave many of the miners pneumonia and fevers. Men who ran out of money slept on the sawdust-covered floors of saloons. Because hygiene was not practiced, indeed was unknown, in the West in those days, and since spitting on the floor of a saloon was accepted practice, these "sawdust gang" miners picked up a variety of diseases. Quinine and whiskey were the common remedies, but this treatment usually hastened pneumonia.

Other diseases, ranging from the common cold to syphilis, were contracted and spread by the "dancehall girls." One such was Nellie Talbott, a woman of pleasure in Bear Town, Montana (Phillips, 1962). Beautiful and cultured, Nellie was bothered by a persistent, hacking cough. A doctor prescribed some medicine and advised her to avoid alternate hot and cold. She took the medicine, but her line of work kept her from following his advice. Nellie had saved a tidy amount of money and could have quit her profession if she had so chosen. Instead, she loaned the money to her husband, an unprincipled man who apparently lacked gratitude, for shortly thereafter he left her. Illness caused Nellie's beauty to fade, and her followers deserted her. She became a scrubwoman and finally died at age sixty of pneumonia in Phillipsburg, Montana.

Scurvy was prevalent in those mining camps, and the people went to imaginative lengths to concoct a home cure. A "mother lode" remedy was to bury the afflicted person in the ground with only his head sticking out. One traveler came across an entire camp "buried" alive, except for a few men who stood guard against marauding grizzlies and coyotes who might be tempted to taste those being "treated."

Silicosis was exceptionally common among the miners, and hardrock miners at Central City, Colorado, died at an average age of 38. Dr. H. A. Lemen of Denver described a silicosis sufferer at one of the first meetings of the Colorado State Medical Society (Dunlop, 1965):

> He was expectorating daily large quantities of fluid, a specimen of which I exhibit you in this bottle. He not infrequently expectorated a pint and a half or two pints of this fluid in 24 hours. His pillow case and shirt bosom were bespattered with what looked like black ink. The sentence that I am now reading was written with this fluid. The pen used has never been in ink.

Neglect or ignorance made many of the afflictions worse. In 1867, Dr. Glick removed a seventy-foot tapeworm from Luke Byrne, a Bear Gulch (Montana) miner who had treated himself with booze and homemade laxatives until he was too weak to dig. About that same time in Summit (Montana), Frank Talty, his wife, his toddler, and visiting neighbors became violently ill one evening after dinner. Dr. Allen Fowler found that Talty had pounded ore and placed it in a pan of mercury to separate the gold. The mercury fumes impregnated the food, poisoning the family and their guests. The adults recovered, but the Talty baby died (Dunlop, 1965).

The Military. Military camps, too, brought men and disease; and accidents followed them into the camps and created need for medical care. Fort Ruby, Nevada, established in 1862, had a stockade-type hospital in which soldiers, settlers, travelers, and even Indians were treated by Army doctors, the first professional medical men in northeastern Nevada.

Treatments at the fort were mostly for malaises brought about by the unstable environmental situation: arrow wounds, broken bones, blisters, frozen hands, and pneumonia. The doctors did what they could, but their knowledge was as limited as their equipment, which consisted mainly of hooks, gouges, mallets, probes, and forceps; and when physicians were at a loss for a cure, amputation was often ordered. Whiskey again was the usual drug; alcohol diluted with carbolic acid, plus soap and water, the accepted antiseptics. To cure those unlucky enough to contract venereal disease, the fort doctors sent entire details of men north to a ranch in Myers, where they sat on stone pots built over hot springs in an attempt to steam away the disease. In 1869, Camp Halleck, eighty miles northwest of Fort Ruby, had outbreaks of malaria, cholera morbus, and diarrhea, due partially to the fact that the privy drained into the water supply. Protection from any disease was indeed not helped by the filthy barracks, poor ventilation, and lice and other vermin that crawled from man to man (Patterson, 1972).

Herb Givers and Bloodletters

Whether a Mormon, a miner, or a military man, many preferred home remedies to a doctor's treatment for a common reason: People were afraid of doctors. With or without medical training, their early treatments were often as harmful as they were helpful. Many patients probably feared the physician's treatment more than the disease itself.

Two major categories of practitioner in early pioneer medicine were the "heroics," those who cured by letting out some of the patient's blood and by administering drugs which caused vomiting and diarrhea, and the "Thomsonians," those who were against bloodletting and swore by herbal treatments. But two other categories existed in the Old West: the eclectics and the quacks (with their curealls). Let us examine these four types of practitioner.

Heroics. The word "heroic" is defined as "daring and risky, but used as a last resort." If anything, heroic medicine was risky! In general, it consisted of bleeding, blistering, purging, and sweating. These treatments were based on the belief (during that time) that the symptoms should be treated, and when the symptom was no longer apparent, the disease was cured.

Kaufman (1971) tells us that bloodletting was "intended to moderate vascular excitement, reduce inflammation, relieve congestion, alleviate spasm and pain, relax muscles and arrest hemorrhage." One of its many firm advocates was Dr. John Milton Bernheisel, who practiced in Utah in the 1850s, and is referred to in records as a "skillful doctor." Rose (1939) states that Bernheisel's belief in the benefits of bleeding were so strong that once, when another doctor protested the amount of blood Bernheisel was drawing, the doctor replied, "Bleed her to death" – meaning "bleed her until she faints." Doctors customarily took from several ounces of blood to several pints, depending upon the ailment and the courage of the physician.

Thomsonians. While many settlers were convinced that the heroic-type treatment was best, bleeding, blistering, and purging were not foolproof. In fact, it was because so many became disgusted with this method that the Thomsonian type of medicine came into being. This method was named for Samuel Thomson, a New Hampshire farmer who blamed heroic practitioners for his mother's death, saying (Rothstein, 1972):

> The doctors gave her over, and gave her disease the name of galloping consumption, which I thought was a very appropriate name; for they are the riders and their whip is mercury, opium, and vitriol, and they galloped her out of this world in about nine weeks.

Later, Thomson's wife became ill after childbirth, and the bleeder's method made her weaker. Thomson dismissed the heroic physician and brought in two herb doctors under whose treatment she recovered. This influenced him to give up his farm to become an herbal doctor himself. By 1811, he had a system of medicine established and had started a lay medical society; by 1813, his plan was patented.

Thomson was not without knowledge of or experience with herbs, however, for he had become interested in herbs and their healing properties when he was four years old and ate lobelia, a milky plant that, when consumed, causes vomiting. This experience to the child was "so remarkable, I never forgot it" (Alter, 1942). He later enjoyed inducing his friends to eat the plant and then watching the consequences. Thomson spent much of his youth observing herb doctors and, despite what seemed to be sadistic childhood tendencies, soon had a reputation as a healer.

Thomson's childhood discovery of lobelia and its peculiarities soon became the mainstay of his followers. One such advocate, Priddy Meeks, a Mormon Thomsonian who believed in witchcraft and cursed the corset as the perpetrator of diseases and deformities in women (saying, "tho slow, it is sure"), said of the flower (Alter, 1942):

> I sometimes look upon lobelia as being supernatural, although I have been using it for 46 years. . . . It is undoubtedly the best and purest relaxum in the compass of medicine. That is the reason it is good in childbed cases; it puts the system in exactly the situation the laws of nature would like to have it be in to perform that object. Those in the habit of using it in such cases look forward in pleasing anticipation of having a good time, without foreboding of trouble so common to women.

While Thomson might have had a set idea as to the causes and cures of disease, his followers used treatments probably more diverse than the illnesses they saw. But like the heroics, Thomsonians evinced resourcefulness that did not always mean success. In the 1870s, Martha Spence Heywood treated her daughter for measles. She bathed the child in saleratus water and gave her tea and sage, all of which were ineffective. She then gave her castor oil followed by lobelia to purge her system of a canker medicine containing blue vitriol that she had given the child earlier. To work off the lobelia that remained, the mother gave the little girl rhubarb, and the child seemed to improve, but then relapsed. In another attempt, onions were put under the child's arms and her feet placed in hot water. By the following day, the child appeared to be dying, and the mother used lobelia again, which brought up phlegm, and the girl seemed relieved. However, the child died on the following day (Larson, 1957).

This exemplifies the "hit and miss" methods of medicine used by pioneers and their doctors. Without any real scientific basis for medical practice and with no diagnostic equipment other than the naked eye, the doctors could do nothing but try one method and, if that failed, try another until, inevitably, the patient either recovered or succumbed to the malady.

Eclectics. A third school of practice was "eclectic" medicine. While it offered itself as an alternative to its two basic predecessors, in reality it couldn't be termed a worthwhile choice. Eclecticism was founded in the 1820s by Wooster Beach, a medical school graduate who also studied with a botanical doctor. Beach was a critic of heroic medicine and turned to all available sources he could find for his ideas, including Thomsonianism and Indian remedies. Because his principles were taken from many sources, he called himself "an eclectic."

Eclectics claimed to be against the use of calomel, a dangerous laxative favored by the heroics, and the abuse of the lancet. They said that they advocated specific medication, the prescribing of certain drugs for certain symptoms. However, they seemed merely to copy heroic medicine, replacing regular drugs with others which produced similar physiological effects.

The Quacks and the Curealls. Pioneers could indeed find good reason to mistrust doctors; yet many seemed to be lured by quackery. "Bill the Healer" was one such charlatan who "practiced" medicine in Wyoming in the 1870s. He and an accomplice traveled from town to town staging their act in order to sell Bill's "magic touch." Their routine went something like this: Bill would enter a saloon where he was of course a stranger; and the accomplice, who had preceded Bill into the place, would feign a strange, debilitating attack. Bill would provide an instant "cure," the news of which quickly spread to the townspeople, bringing patients with a variety of diseases – and money. Bill and his accomplice would then move on to another town.

Others were lured by the promises of patent medicines – such as the "King of Pain," a concoction that was touted as being good for baldness, and if that wasn't the problem, then it would be beneficial for deafness as well. Selling patent medicine became a prosperous enterprise in the Old West because the settlers were often ignorant of medicines and wanted a quick, inexpensive way to good health. In addition, because there were not enough doctors for all of the settlements, the claims of the medicine hawkers added excitement to a harsh and dreary existence. Besides, the contents of these medicines could be enticing. For example, Colden's Liquid Beef Tonic, similar to many others of that era, offered itself as a treatment for those addicted to alcohol, and it contained 26.5 percent of the stuff!

Epidemic in Any Case

With or without medical care, the early pioneers seemed to contract and die from a variety of diseases. Epidemics often were rampant because no one knew what caused the sickness. Quarantines were of course unheard of. Of all the dread diseases, smallpox was the most feared. One of the worst epidemics occurred in 1869 when the steamer "Utah" came upriver to Fort Benton, Montana, with several crew members ill of the disease. One of the men died before the fort was reached and was buried on the banks of the Milk River. The Gros Ventre Indians discovered the grave and dug up the corpse for its clothing. They not only fell ill of the disease but also became carriers, infecting the entire tribe with smallpox. It is estimated that eight hundred of the fifteen hundred members of that tribe died from this one episode. As was their custom, the Gros Ventres placed their dead in trees, and white traders filched the skin robes and sold them, thus spreading the epidemic even farther (Phillips, 1962).

In 1868 an outbreak of smallpox among Nevada workers on the Central Pacific Railroad caused a daily mortality rate of three to five. So many died that the bodies were loaded onto railroad cars and taken to a gulch two miles west of Elko. The gulch became a common, unmarked grave for these people.

Smallpox was so severe in territorial Wyoming that one of the only two laws there concerning health dealt with the disease, making it a misdemeanor to intentionally spread smallpox. The other law concentrated on the handling of "lunatics... and the habitual drunk" (Huebert, 1962).

In retrospect, one must note that this disease need not have been such a killer, for Edward Jenner, who developed and first used his vaccine in 1796, had made it available to the entire populace. But many of the Westerners were as afraid of the vaccination as they were of the disease.

Vaccination. The closing years of the nineteenth century in Utah found smallpox so common that surrounding states complained that Utah was a source of danger to the entire Intermountain West. Utah newspapers carried daily reports of outbreaks and deaths from the disease. Dr. Theodore B. Beatty, then state health commissioner, recommended to the board of health that vaccination for smallpox be made compulsory because the disease was so widespread that the situation was becoming more and more intolerable.

The reaction of the citizenry was intensely anti-vaccination. For it to become compulsory was declared unconstitutional, "a loss of personal rights," some said. Others spread tales of blood poisonings and loss of legs, arms, and life due to vaccination. And there was a possibility of secondary infection. For example, in Nevada, when some of the earliest health legislation in that state provided for the distribution of vaccine, there was little supervision, and sometimes a scab would be taken from one town to another where families would be "vaccinated." But infection was generally an overrated danger. Yet many were frightened by tales of the disease and would rather run the risk of contracting smallpox than introduce it into their bodies with vaccine.

The opposition was soon organized round the editorials of the *Deseret News*, and since it was the official paper of the LDS church, many believed that the church was against vaccination, and hostility intensified. Anti-vaccination editorials appeared frequently for almost a year. However, according to Morrell (1956), officials of the church made no statement against vaccination. In fact, George Q. Cannon, former editor of the *Deseret News* and at that time serving as first councilor to President Lorenzo Snow, had written favorably of vaccination in an editorial many years before. He had told of the benefits as well as the alleged dangers. In summary, he had said: "If the evidence can be relied upon, vaccination is an excellent preventive, and people should avail themselves of it as a guard against smallpox."

Another voice in favor of vaccination had been raised as early as 1888 by the paper *Woman's Exponent*, the official voice of the LDS women's organization called the "Relief Society" (Morrell, 1956):

> This is a subject which, by us as a people, is much neglected, and there is a great deal of prejudice against it, perhaps not without much cause. But if someone who understands would take the interest in it, and attend to it in the proper way, there need be no fear of transmitting disease from one to another.

Morrell feels that the editorial opposition to vaccination can be traced to the fact that the *Deseret News* editor had grown up in England where compulsory vaccination had been forced and had provoked dissidence because Britons thought it a violation of human rights. Before coming to America, this man had been an editorial writer for the *Millennial Star*, a publication of the LDS branch of the church in England, and had written many anti-vaccination editorials for that paper.

Dr. Beatty campaigned vigorously for vaccination, telling of the million vaccinations in New York which had not produced adverse results, and in 1901 he offered a reward of $1,000 to anyone in Utah who could prove the loss of an arm because of vaccination. Armed with data on Utah's abysmal smallpox record, Beatty went before the state legislature to argue for the law. The legislators, however, saw fit to enact the McMillan bill, which repealed the compulsory vaccination ordinance and branded the board of health as "a useless agency, expensive to the state, and wholly incompetent.... [T]hey [agency members] were led by a dictatorial Health Commissioner and had no independent minds" (Morrell, 1956). Governor Heber H. Wells promptly vetoed the bill, and just as swiftly it was passed over his veto, an action generally celebrated throughout the state.

The celebration would not have taken place if the people had but realized that vaccination is a sound preventive measure. During the 1920s and '30s, smallpox was almost eradicated in several states because of compulsory vaccination; but it still prevailed in Utah which, many claim, had more cases of smallpox than any other state.

The rate of smallpox cases per hundred thousand population in Utah can be compared with other states in Table 1-1. At the time that this information was published in 1936, compulsory vaccination was prohibited in Utah and Wisconsin had no compulsory vaccination, but New York and Massachusetts had compulsory vaccination.

Spotted Fever. Rocky Mountain spotted fever was another mysterious and deadly disease that some claimed came from drinking melted snow and others said lived in sawdust. No one really knew what caused this wretched disease, but everyone who had come into contact with it knew that it could turn a robust young person into a ruddy-colored corpse within a matter of a few days.

Montana's Bitter Root Valley, ten miles wide and fifty miles long, was most severely afflicted with the disease. The valley, covered in the early spring with the pink blossoms of the plant for which it is named, was home to settlers who lived in fear of Rocky Mountain spotted fever. While the bitterroot was commonly used as an herbal medicine, it was no cure for spotted fever. Cold baths could relieve the patient's discomfort because of the high fever that

Table 1-1

Case Rate of Smallpox per Hundred Thousand Population in Four States

(Selected years)

	Rate of Smallpox Cases			
Year	Utah	Wisconsin	New York	Massachusetts
1920	1,131.2	124.2	2.9	0.7
1925	23.5	54.2	2.5	0.1
1930	24.6	32.4	2.6	0.0
1935	7.4	22.3	0.0	0.0

is characteristic of the disease, but, as one doctor said (Aikawa, 1966), "In general, the therapeutic measures should be directed toward conserving the strength of the patient... thus insuring the most favorable circumstances for the natural forces of the body against infection."

In March 1901, Montana established a state board of health, and the governor gave the board's secretary, Dr. A. F. Longeway, his first assignment: Do something about spotted fever. "I have just had an appeal from the people of the Bitter Root," the governor told Longeway (Price, 1948). The doctor was given $2,000 to work with (an amount that easily could have been spent educating the populace about vaccination – for smallpox was rampant in Montana – or against unlicensed embalmers, or for typhoid fever and the state's lack of sanitation measures). But Longeway decided that Rocky Mountain spotted fever rated first priority. He asked Dr. Earle Strain from Great Falls for help, and the two men went to Missoula and Stevensville in the Bitter Root country to investigate the "black measles," as spotted fever was often called.

It was not hard to find several recent victims of the disease. Strain noticed ticks on the bulging bodies and remembered medical lectures on the mosquito and its role as a carrier of yellow fever. He suggested ticks were the cause, but the idea was laughed at. Ticks? No, it's the melted snow, he was told. That's why it was so common among sheepherders and stockmen who went up into the mountains in the early spring and had nothing else to drink.

Dr. Longeway asked the board of health of Minnesota for extra help, and in May 1902, a pathologist, Dr. Louis B. Wilson, arrived, followed by Dr. William Chowning. Their investigations found that the first case in the Bitter Root was in May of 1873, and was fatal, as were 80 percent of the two hundred other cases on record. It was its high mortality, not high incidence, that made it so feared. On the other side of the mountain in Idaho, the disease was less severe and did not always kill. Of 114 cases they documented, most occurred in ranchers and timber cruisers who went into the foothills, or to their families. More men than women were afflicted. In one month, Wilson and Chowning saw seven healthy persons die of Rocky Mountain spotted fever – all of whom had been bitten by a tick. This, plus the fact that most of the victims had occupations that took them into the tick-infested foothills, made the tick a possibility indeed.

In 1904, Wilson and Chowning did not return to resume their studies, for the Montana Board of Health was preoccupied with a typhoid epidemic that stretched nearly three hundred miles from Bozeman to Milk River. Many people were pleased that the investigation was halted. While western Montana was full of productive orchards and dairy herds, it was still sparsely settled. Special trains brought prospective buyers from outside, and if they were to hear about spotted fever, large amounts of money might be lost to those involved in real estate. Besides, it just wasn't comfortable to believe the tick theory; people could dig wells and avoid the mountain water in the spring, but it was difficult to keep away from the ticks.

Dr. Ricketts Arrives. Dr. Howard Ricketts, from the University of Chicago, decided in 1906 that he would take up the Rocky Mountain spotted fever study on his own accord, and he proved invaluable to the research. Ricketts demonstrated that a tick who fed on a guinea pig ill of the fever could transmit the disease to a healthy pig. The same experiment was also successful with monkeys and it was now certain that the tick was the carrier of the infection.

The Montana State Legislature was so impressed with Rickett's work that in 1909 it appropriated $6,000 for his studies. But when the board of examiners found that various appropriations had exceeded the state treasury, it trimmed the budget by cutting out medical research, telling Ricketts the money was not available. The funds were finally released in December, and Ricketts, who by this time had accepted an invitation to study typhus in Mexico, said he would try to be in Montana by May 1, 1910.

But Ricketts never made it back. He contracted typhus and died May 3, 1910. By now several others were committed to the cause, including Willard King, a student at Montana State University who worked for the U.S. Bureau of Entomology, and Clarence Birdseye, an Amherst College student and field naturalist for the U.S. Biological Survey in the West, who, on a later study in the arctic, developed the idea of frozen foods.

A farm was rented three miles southwest of Florence, in the heart of the Bitter Root, and a laboratory set up in a log cabin whose previous occupant had died of Rocky Mountain spotted fever just one year before. The researchers planned to study the tick and its life cycle, and the farm proved an excellent place, for ticks were crawling all over the yard. King, Birdseye, and the others with them decided to sleep out-of-doors, so the yard was burned and then sprayed with oil. As a further precaution, a camp rule was made that every two hours, no matter what they were doing, the men were to strip and inspect themselves for ticks.

Despite dangers and inconvenience, the studies proved fruitful. It was discovered that grown ticks attached themselves to large animals, where they not only fed but mated, while the younger insects fed on small rodents such as gophers. If this feeding could be prevented, the ticks would die, or at least diminish in number. Dipping horses and cattle in oil would eliminate many adult ticks, while shooting gophers would kill those in the younger stages.

Tick Control Established. Three Montana tick control districts which required dipping of animals were established in 1913, but the program had many snags. At first there was a delay in rounding up the cattle; by the time they were corralled, the water and kerosene mixture used as a dip had separated, subjecting the cows to almost pure oil and burning their udders. Once the dip was too strong and burned hides. Another time, good grazing grass was killed by drippings off the animals. Some cows would drop in milk production, or were even killed by the dip. A safe formula was finally developed, but by this time so had hostility, and during 1914 one vat was wrecked with a crow bar and another dynamited.

By the end of the season, however, the tick population had definitely been reduced and there were fewer cases of spotted fever. Without the blood-sucking ticks, animals were healthier, too; and by the fall of 1915, even the most antagonistic farmer had a hard time refuting the value of tick control measures.

Another major advancement was made in 1919 when a professor of pathology at Harvard Medical School, S. Burt Wolbach, found the causative agent of the disease. Then in the early 1920s Drs. R. R. Parker and R. R. Spencer of the U.S. Public Health Service started their search for a vaccine. They developed one made from adult ticks collected in the field, a dangerous, tedious, and expensive process. The captured ticks were allowed to feed on guinea pigs that had just come down with the disease. After two days of feeding, the ticks were stored for several months, then fed on normal animals for five or six days, ground with mortar and pestle and added to a preservative of 1.6 percent phenol and 0.4 percent formalin. Spencer made the first test of this vaccine on himself (Aikawa, 1966).

In the spring of 1925, there was only enough vaccine for 34 persons in the Bitter Root Valley. It was to be given in two doses at five day intervals and cost $20 an injection.

The first vaccination program was carried out in 1926 in both the Bitter Root Valley and in Idaho. It proved to be very successful. In the Bitter Root, the mortality rate was lowered and the period of illnesses shortened; and in Idaho there was one case of Rocky Mountain spotted fever among the vaccinated group and 22 cases among the same number of unvaccinated volunteers.

Success was so promising that in 1927 the Montana State Legislature was requested to fund a new building for the state board of entomology and in 1928, the Montana Research Laboratory in Hamilton came into being. Here tick cultivation was started on a large scale. At the peak more than a million infected ticks were cultivated in one year, which required fifteen thousand to twenty thousand guinea pigs and six thousand rabbits (Aikawa, 1966).

In 1930 the federal government bought the lab and took over production of the vaccine. The new Rocky Mountain research lab developed a less dangerous method and increased production; by 1948 it could produce enough serum for 140,000 people at $1.00 an injection. It was none too soon, says Price (1948), for also by 1948, only six states – Maine, Vermont, Rhode Island, Connecticut, Michigan, and Kansas – had not reported cases of the once mysterious and deadly Rocky Mountain spotted fever.

Typhoid. Prior to 1900, local doctors saw more typhoid fever than any other disease. They treated it in various ways; some felt it was best to starve the patient, others felt hot water was the cure. Typhoid was prevalent in the railroad camps, one Nevada camp having 47 victims hospitalized at one time.

But no one person or place was exempt. In Salt Lake City, 925 deaths listed in the cemetery books from 1850 to 1894 are recorded as due to typhoid, but the actual number was probably even higher, according to Richards (1953). Many of the deaths among typhoid-prone adolescents and young adults, who died in the summer and autumn when typhoid is most common, were simply attributed to "diarrhea" or "fever."

Typhoid entered the body through bacteria on food and drink and was easy enough to contract, for early sanitation practices were scarce. Shallow wells often caught drainage from corrals and barnyards, and in Nevada for many years sewer lines discharged directly into the rivers. Food and milk inspectors were still in the future, and people could not resist the temptation to lie down and drink drainage ditch water which looked clear and tasted cold, but in which typhoid germs from nearby privies often proliferated.

Many persons realized the connection between typhoid and contaminated food and drink, but little action was taken until health boards were established. Even then, it was difficult to impress upon people how a few precautions could prevent many needless deaths. Also, the attitude of "what was good enough for my grandfather is good enough for me" was common, said Mustard (1936), and "when grandfather used a fence corner rather than a sanitary privy, the disciple of sanitation finds himself battling with custom and tradition."

Salt Lake City was a hotbed for typhoid, as were many other U.S. cities during the late nineteenth and early twentieth centuries. People would hunt, camp, picnic, and pollute near the seven mountain streams that provided the city with most of its water. Sheep and cattle would graze near the watershed, barnyards were built near water sources, and flies had easy access to the open privies and manure piles.

"Swat the Fly." When the housefly was implicated as a typhoid carrier about the time of the Spanish-American War, Dr. Beatty began a crusade against the pest. He distributed literature, gave talks and demonstrations at schools, and helped make "Swat the Fly" become a common greeting. A contest was even set up whereby prizes were offered to whoever killed the most flies. The

winner of first place, which was $1,000 donated by a Salt Lake City businessman, brought in 707 quarts of dead flies, an estimated 9.5 million. In one year, Utahns captured 3,715 quarts of flies for the health department. The fly menace was lessened; but real progress was made when attention gradually turned to the eradication of breeding places (Morrell, 1956).

Several eastern cities had tried chlorinating their water as protection against typhoid, with good results. Following this example, Salt Lake City instituted a program of chlorination in 1915, adding to it until 1927 when daily testing of chlorinated water was done at all city water intake points. It was then found that the chlorine mixture was not constant or adequate enough to control the baccilli, and corrective measures were undertaken, also with good results. Data on the results of chlorination are as follows (Richards, 1953):

Time and Kind of Chlorination Treatment	*Annual Average Typhoid Cases*
Six years before chlorination in 1915 (untreated)	220.0
Six years of partial chlorination (1915 to 1920)	79.0
Six years of all-year chlorination (1921 to 1926, no controls; serious food epidemic in 1924)	69.0
Eight years of controlled chlorine dosage (1927 to 1934; in 1930, ammonia was added, making it more effective)	26.0
Seven years (1935 to 1941)	3.5

No typhoid was reported from 1942 until Richards' book was printed in 1953.

Reactions to the addition of chlorine in the water were varied. The board of health heard from worried mothers who couldn't taste the chlorine and wondered if the water were safe. Others alleged that chlorine made the water unpalatable. Furthermore, the chlorine killed their goldfish; but, worst of all in these prohibition days, it ruined the taste of their "home brew" and their bathtub gin.

Typhoid was also easily passed by finger contamination when an ill person or even a recovered victim handled food and didn't wash his or her hands carefully after using the toilet. Richards told in his book how tragic such a situation might be. In 1923 a Salt Lake City woman working in a delicatessen was ill with what was later diagnosed as "walking typhoid." She had diarrhea and was getting weaker, but didn't want to leave her boss shorthanded; besides, she needed the money. So she stayed on the job, serving food in between her frequent trips to the lavatory and her not-so-frequent or thorough handwashings.

Meanwhile, a group of six people, four adults and two young people, came to the city from their farm on the west side to see a double feature movie. Afterwards they decided they would be too tired to fix a meal, so they went into the deli and bought some cold food. At home, the two youngsters had dates and left; the adults stayed and ate supper. All four of them came down with typhoid and two died.

A total of 188 cases of typhoid (thirteen deaths) was traced to the woman carrier, but no one knows for sure how many people contracted the disease, took it home, possibly to another state, and spread it even farther. The problem was compounded by the fact that a drugstore near Salt Lake's tourist section bought food from the delicatessen and served it to uncounted numbers of people. Eventually the deli was tracked down and quarantined, and the epidemic subsided.

With increasing use of sanitary methods – improved sewer systems, purer water, and laws regulating the handling and dispensing of foods – plus use of a vaccine discovered by Almoth Wright of London in 1906–07 – typhoid was eventually controlled.

Diphtheria. Incidence of diphtheria mushroomed as families with children filtered into the area; by 1876 it was a genuine problem. Easily transmitted by clothing, dishes, or any personal contact, it was once suggested in 1896 by the *Deseret News* that doctors' beards were the culprits. This contagion was not helped by the fact that parents seemed oblivious to the dangers, allowing well children to play with the sick and continue to attend school during epidemics. Salt Lake City faced an especially harsh bout with diphtheria in 1879 when 178 deaths were reported, and two to five deaths in a single week in one family were not uncommon.

In Wyoming, Miss Martha Jane Canary, better known as Calamity Jane, reportedly nursed a little girl who had "black diphtheria," which is what the frontier people called the child killer. A youngster's only protection against it, and many of the other childhood diseases, was often a bag of asafetida and camphor tied round his or her neck.

Respiratory Ailments. Harsh winters spurred many respiratory ailments, and pneumonia became a seasonal killer of large numbers of people. Teamsters hauling freight across the frozen Nevada desert, cowboys, ranchers, miners, anyone who had to brave the cold, all were vulnerable, despite the whiskey used to "warm the innards."

During the American pioneer period, tuberculosis was a perilous threat throughout the world. Many consumptive immigrants from England's industrial centers came to the mines of Utah, and other tuberculars traveled to the West hoping that the climate would be beneficial for their condition. One of these was John Henry Holliday, an Atlanta gentleman and dentist usually remembered as gun-slinging Doc Holliday. Besides being a tubercular, Holliday was a nervous individual who once confessed to Wyatt Earp that he was calm only while fighting or working on teeth. He ultimately succumbed to the disease in Glenwood Springs, Colorado.

Unsanitary practices spread tuberculosis (TB) to many people. As late as 1906, a Dr. Tuttle wrote (Phillips, 1962):

> The floors of the day coaches [of trains] are covered with all kinds of filth. The tobacco chewer spits on the floor, the little boy throws his peanut hulls on the floor, the consumptive expectorates on the floor. All this filth and trash accumulates until the division point is reached, then comes the brakeman with this broom.... He is anxious not to lose a minute at the end of his run, and he brushed this dread filth into a dust that is simply stifling; and this dust is laden with the germs of tuberculosis. The passengers must breath it; they cannot get away from it; they cannot get out of the car, and the law says they must not kill the brakeman.

Mining and Health

The period from 1872 to 1892 saw a phenomenal development in western mining – which brought with it a plethora of health problems. Pollution from the smelters, for example, could become extremely high. In Eureka, Nevada (almost every state had its

"Eureka!" – meaning "I have found it!" in Greek), pollution was so severe that it killed all of the cats. But nowhere in the United States was lead poisoning, which can lead to local paralysis or collapse, as bad as it was in Utah. According to Richards (1953):

> In the days when lead poisoning was most prevalent, the miners worked twelve hours a day underground. No baths were systematically taken for cleanliness; there was no forced ventilation to remove the dust. The clothes worn by the workers became impregnated with lead ore dust and were seldom changed. Under those conditions the victim was exposed to lead absorption twenty-four hours a day and frequently succumbed to poisoning. The smelter workers were not only exposed to dust, but in addition were placed in contact with lead fumes that were equally liable to absorption through the skin.

Dust and fumes were also inhaled, passed into the body's circulatory system, and distributed to all of the organs.

The standard treatment for lead poisoning – or "plumbism," as it was called – was a saturated salt solution with tincture of iron, a half-ounce per gallon, and with a little oil of wintergreen for flavoring. A tablespoonful or more was given to make the patient become thirsty so that he would drink copious amounts of water. When the water was eliminated, the poison was to go with it, in theory. But since modern medical expertise was unavailable, there is no record of how many died from the poisoning or the cure.

Early Hospitals in the Intermountain West

Mining not only had its lead poisoning problems, it also brought more accidents to the Intermountain Area. Although accidents had become a way of life to the hardy frontier settlers – usually entailing broken bones – with the advent of mining in the region, accidents tended to accelerate, and mining accidents could be more serious. There were bonesetters in nearly every area, but trained medical practitioners were few. And there were no hospitals.

In 1872, the Episcopal church helped establish a small adobe hospital in Salt Lake City, St. Mark's, the first in the Utah Territory. It was financed in part by mining companies which paid a subscription for the care of their employees. The miners contributed $1.00 each per month; this entitled them to a bed in St. Mark's and care while they were confined there. For several years, more than 50 percent of the admissions to the hospital were "leaded," reaching to 67 percent in one particular year.

The addition of such a facility did not mean that all was well with medicine in the Intermountain West (Behle, 1948). When Miss Mary Newitt became superintendent of the training school for nurses at St. Mark's in 1894, she found conditions there abominable (yet they were typical of all but the most modern hospitals of the time). Dirt was in abundance everywhere. One patient, recently operated upon, had no clean sheets because a nursing attendant had quit and no one had bothered to check on whether she had completed her assigned duties before she left.

The operating room had no facilities for sterilization, and several cuspidors under the operating table (whose leather top was soaked with blood) were filled with dirty dressings. Multitudes of flies infested the hospital by day and mosquitoes by night. Miss Newitt determined that the hospital must be cleaned up and set out to improve conditions. According to Behle (1948):

> She had the cuspidors, sheets, and upholstered leather table top buried in the back yard of the hospital. She obtained some boards and constructed a new table top that could be scrubbed. The legs of the table were scrubbed and painted. This operating table was used for many months. Clean blankets and sheets were placed on top for each operation. With the help of several scrub women, the whole hospital was finally cleaned up.

A few other hospitals were built during the late 1800s, but many of the sick were kept in their homes, or perhaps in a room of the doctor's house. In those days, according to Walker (1944), families preferred not going to a hospital, for they felt it was tantamount to "a death sentence. Such hospitals as they knew or had heard of were uninviting – poor beds, poor nursing, and food uninviting – and worse yet, they were deprived of the sympathy and loving care of family and friends."

Pest Houses. Impoverished citizens with contagious diseases were sent to a "pest house" – generally a cabin on the outskirts of the town, by law at least a mile from the nearest dwelling. If the snow happened to be deep, the sheriff would escort the afflicted "outcast" only so far and then give him a key and tell him to make himself "at home." The patient was expected to prepare his own meals (from food he himself had provided), take care of his own needs, and supply his own bedding and other essentials.

Stewards from the county's "poor house" were to look in on these abject souls occasionally and a physician was to check on them each day, but many were found dead from lack of continuous and proper care.

Other Early Hospitals. One of the first hospitals in the Intermountain Area was built in Bannock City, Idaho (now Idaho City). Funds for the hospital were supplied by the Boise County Commissioners in the autumn of 1863, and three doctors – Harris, Crane, and Terry – agreed that for $34 a week they would provide medical care, nursing, and board to each patient. Sick prisoners in the county jail were also covered under these terms.

In Montana, a hospital for Indians was established by the Sisters of Charity of Providence in the St. Ignatius Mission. To them, "healing was a divine duty and was to prepare the Indians for healing of their spiritual life" (Phillips, 1962). To keep the Indians from backsliding to "savagery" and the influence of their medicine men, an infirmary was set up in one room of a house. When this room became filled with sick Indians, one could always see a "sick ring" of teepees outside the home. The Sisters diagnosed common ailments, set bones, and did minor surgery. To get funds for their needed equipment, they often went on begging trips to Oregon and Washington (Phillips, 1962).

St. John's Hospital was Montana's first well-equipped general hospital. It was located in Helena, the state's most populous city and its medical center for a length of time. Completed in 1873, St. John's grew rapidly, and a much larger building was erected in 1874. The new hospital included rooms for the care of the insane.

Creation of a six-bed hospital in Elko County, Nevada, in 1869 was deemed necessary because of a severe outbreak of smallpox at that time. A statute made it mandatory to distribute smallpox vaccine and gave responsibility to look after the poor who were ill to the county commissioners. As a result, when Elko County was established on March 5, 1869, a provision was made for erecting a county indigent hospital and a pest house. Many of the thousands of Chinese who had worked on the transcontinental railroad, which was completed that year, were virtually stranded in the West, and hundreds of them settled in Elko. But Chinese indigents were not allowed treatment at Elko County Hospital (since it was funded by citizens' taxes and therefore could not care for non-citizens), thus another facility came into being – the Elko Chinese Hospital. Although its facilities were crude, the Chinese physicians were highly skilled. Drs. Ken Fung and Long Yut were the first physicians to staff the hospital; both were graduates of China's Canton School of Medicine and Surgery. These physicians, along with Chinese herb doctors, relied on natural drugs and their own training (Patterson, 1972).

One creditable effort to establish a hospital began in Reno, Nevada, in 1904. Dr. J. L. Robinson and associates had organized the "People's Hospital Association" and had leased and cleaned a large building, furnishing it with modern medical equipment. They grew ambitious for a better facility and purchased lots near a school and started to sell stock, but the neighborhood residents didn't favor a hospital next door. A politician in the group got the state legislature to enact a law that would preclude the building of a hospital within five hundred feet of a school, and the plans had to be dropped.

The first Wyoming hospitals were those maintained by the U.S. Army for the use of troops while Wyoming was still a territory. There was always a building at the forts and in the camps which was used for a post hospital. The medical officer at Camp Pilot Butte described his facility by saying (Huebert, 1962):

> ...[T]he hospital is a small building divided by a narrow hall; having on one side the ward dispensary and a small storeroom; on the other [were] a stewards' room, sleeping rooms for two men, dining room and kitchen; a lavatory room has recently been added to the back of the building....[T]he ward is 21 x 28 feet...and contains six beds.

Cheyenne was the home of the first Wyoming public hospital, set up in 1867 in a tent. In 1869 a wooden two-story building was erected, the top floor of which was used for a hospital. In 1882 a brick building was constructed which subsequently became the city-county hospital of Laramie County.

The final quarter of the nineteenth century saw a hospital building boom in the Intermountain Region. The boom slowed somewhat in the early 1890s when the nation was suffering from a depression and the price of silver and copper was low, but construction picked up again at the end of the century. As medical men and women started working together in hospitals, and as the practice of medicine became a profession rather than a dalliance by those bent on making money by chicanery, physicians came to see the value of organizing so that they could acquire new knowledge of medicine as it became available throughout the world. But perhaps their greatest accomplishment was to regulate the practice of medicine in their own states.

Medical Societies

Medical societies have existed in the United States since 1766 when the first was organized in a New Jersey tavern. But those were turbulent times, and physicians soon found the Revolutionary War to be a more pressing matter. The first medical society in the Intermountain Region got off to a slow start. In 1860 several doctors from a part of Colorado called "Jefferson Territory" attempted to organize the Jefferson Medical Society. This was stopped by another war – between the North and South – that claimed their attention. There is no documented evidence that other attempts were made until 1864, when several doctors met at the office of Dr. E. C. Gehrung to establish the Denver Medical Society and agree on a fee schedule (*Medical Coloradoana*, 1922). Gehrung's guests had barely departed when a violent explosion ripped open the gunsmith's shop next door. Gehrung's office was also destroyed, and fire from the gunsmith's shop soon engulfed the doctor's quarters, spreading quickly with the aid of specimen jars containing alcohol that were scattered about the room. As the doctor fought to free himself from the debris and ran to the drugstore for burn medicine, he was seen by several onlookers who misunderstood his gyrations and commented on "that fool running through the fire." This spectacular beginning fizzled into a few more meetings, but must have declined into an inauspicious demise, for there are no records of the society's having survived, and even the records of the follow-up meetings are not in existence.

A second attempt seven years later by other physicians was successful, however, according to the *Medical Coloradoana*, which relates the following story. Several Denver physicians got together "to talk over matters of interest to the profession." This group, the Denver Medical Association, soon sponsored a convention to interest other Colorado doctors in establishing a territorial medical association. In September 1871 the society was formed, with objectives stated as follows:

> ...the improvement of its members in scientific and professional knowledge; the association of the profession for the purpose of mutual recognition and fellowship; the promotion of the character, interest, and honor of the fraternity by maintaining union and harmony, and by aiming to elevate the standard of medical education.

A Dr. Buckingham, president of the Denver Association, gave the address at that historic meeting, closing it with, "May the time soon come that the Territorial Medical Association of Colorado will rest upon as firm a basis as the grand old mountain before us, that lifts its snow-capped summits to the clouds."

The first meetings were devoted to scientific reports, especially those on tuberculosis (or "phthisis," as it was called at that time) and the effect that Colorado's climate had upon it. By 1876, the year that Colorado became a state and the medical society a state institution, there were 51 members.

Nevada's Medical Association. Nevada's first attempt to start a state medical organization was in 1875 (Walker, 1944), but interest soon died because doctors in the Nevada Territory were widely scattered and roads were nonexistent or so primitive that they became impassable in stormy weather. Interest was not reborn until 1904 when state officials realized that the state's tax regulations had attracted a host of quacks within its borders. By then, Reno had gained city status and city fathers were forced to cope with such health problems as garbage and sewage disposal and making sure that the water supply was not contaminated by impurities.

The first annual meeting of the Nevada State Medical Society was in Reno on May 6, 1905. The twenty members who attended the meeting discussed the use of quinine as a cure for pneumonia (at that time, one of Nevada's most killing diseases). A revolutionary idea for that period of time was also discussed – more fresh air for those who were ill. Until then, it had been thought that cold air in the sick room would make pneumonia sufferers even more ill, and all windows and doors were tightly closed and blankets heaped upon the hapless patients. Poultices on throats and chests at all times were prescribed.

The medical society's second year coincided with the year of the San Francisco earthquake. Reno doctors organized themselves into relief committees with headquarters at the train station, where they met and treated trainloads of refugees for shock and, later, for the numerous cases of typhoid and smallpox that broke out after the disaster. Many California physicians had lost their equipment in shattered and burned office buildings, and the Reno doctors donated items of equipment so that the San Francisco doctors could make a new start.

Organized Medicine in Utah. According to the Utah State Medical Association, the first permanent medical society in Utah was begun on February 26, 1895, following an influx of competent, well-trained physicians into the Salt Lake area in the latter part of the century. At the initial meeting of 47 or 49 doctors (accounts vary) the decision was made to elect permanent officers (Bowman, 1969, which quotes the Salt Lake *Tribune,* February 27, 1895):

> ...[The suggestion] brought Dr. Maclean to his feet with a query as to who was eligible to vote for such officers.... "There is one man in the room," Dr. Maclean added, "who is certainly not eligible, and I think he should have had sense enough to have kept away." It was then moved that a committee of three on credentials be appointed, but the motion was not seconded, and it was subsequently decided that all physicians who had received invitations were eligible to cast ballots. Dr. Maclean – "Well, the man I had reference to did not receive an invitation, for I sent them out myself and did not send him one."

The "outcast" on whom Dr. Maclean vent his wrath is not identified. The physicians eventually selected Dr. F. S. Bascom as president, but when it came time to elect a secretary, there was an apparent stuffing of the ballot box (Bowman, 1969):

> ...On the sixth ballot, there were fifty-one ballots cast, and as there were only forty-nine physicians present, the entire vote was thrown out. Some of the members suggested that there were some Democrats present who had stuffed the box,

> and Dr. Maclean arose to inquire if there was a member of the Utah Commission present.... Another ballot was then taken, which resulted in the election of Dr. J. N. Harrison.... At the conclusion of the meeting, as reported by the Salt Lake *Tribune*, Dr. Bascom thanked the society for the honor which they had conferred upon him, and gave evidence of his appreciation by ordering a box of cigars for the male members and a glass of lemonade for Mrs. Dr. Miles, the only lady physician present.

The distinction made between the men ("Dr.") and the "lady physician" ("Mrs. Dr.") was common in those days; and the use of the word "lady" was complimentary, or so the men thought.

Selected References

Aikawa, Jerry K. *Rocky Mountain Spotted Fever*. Springfield, Illinois: Charles C Thomas, Publisher. 1966.

Alter, J. Cecil. Editor. *Utah Historical Quarterly* (1942), vol. x.

Beal, Merrill D.; and Wells, Merle W. "The Gem State, 1890–1956: Economic and Political Maturity." In *History of Idaho*. New York: Lewis Historical Publishing Co., Inc. 1949.

Behle, William H. *Biography of Augustus C. Behle*. Salt Lake City: Private printing. 1948.

Bowman, Harold, "The Organization of the Utah State Medical Association." Salt Lake City: Utah State Medical Association. 1969. Unpublished document.

Collier's Encyclopedia. Volume 20. New York: Cromwell-Collier Educational Corp. 1971.

Colorado State Medical Society. *Medical Coloradoana*. Denver: Colorado State Medical Society. 1922.

Deseret News, Salt Lake City, September 18, 1852.

Divett, Robert T. "Medicine and the Mormons." Salt Lake City: University of Utah's Marriott Library, analytic file. No date. Unpublished manuscript.

Drury, Clifford. *Marcus and Narcissa Whitman.* Glendale, California: The Arthur H. Clark Company. 1973.

Dunlop, Richard. "Medics of the Mining Camps." In *Doctors of the American Frontier.* Garden City, New York: Doubleday & Company Inc. 1965.

Encyclopedia of World Biography. Volume 11. New York: McGraw-Hill Book Company. 1973.

Huebert, Helen M. "Health Needs and Services in Wyoming." Laramie: University of Wyoming. 1962.

Journal of Discourses. Volume 15. Salt Lake City, LDS Church Historian's Office, 1873.

Karolevitz, Robert F. *Doctors of the Old West.* Seattle, Washington: Superior Publishing Co. 1967.

Kaufman, Martin. *Hemeopathy in America.* Baltimore, Maryland: Johns Hopkins University Press. 1971.

Larson, Andrew Carl. *The Red Hills of November.* Salt Lake City: The Deseret News Press. 1957.

Markley, Arthur J. "The Colorado State Medical Society: In Retrospect on the 76th Anniversary of Its Organization." *Rocky Mountain Medical Journal* (December 1946).

Morrell, Joseph R. *Utah's Health and You: A History of Utah's Public Health.* Salt Lake City: Deseret Book Company. 1956.

Mustard, Harry S. *Rural Health Practice.* New York: The Commonwealth Fund. 1936.

Myers, John. *Doc Holliday.* Boston, Massachusetts: Little, Brown and Company. 1955.

Patterson, Edna B. *Sagebrush Doctors.* Springville, Utah: Art City Publishing Co. 1972.

Phillips, Paul C. *Medicine in the Making of Montana.* Missoula: Montana State University Press. 1962.

Price, Esther G. *Fighting Spotted Fever in the Rockies.* Helena, Montana: Naegele Printing Co. 1948.

Richards, Ralph T. "History of Medicine in Utah." *Bulletin of the University of Utah* (June 1946), vol. 36, no. 15.

———. *Of Medicine, Hospitals and Doctors.* Salt Lake City: University of Utah Press. 1953.

Rose, Blanche. "The History of Medicine in Utah." Salt Lake City: University of Utah. 1939. Master's thesis.

Rothstein, William G. *American Physicians in the Nineteenth Century*. Baltimore, Maryland: Johns Hopkins University Press. 1972.

Salt Lake *Tribune*, February 27, 1895.

Utah State Planning Committee. *Health Conditions and Facilities in Utah*. Salt Lake City: Utah State Planning Committee. 1936.

Walker, M. R. *Life's Review and Notes on the Development of Medicine in Nevada, 1900–1944*. Second revision. Reno, Nevada: Private printing. 1944.

2

From the Dark Ages — A Quickening

"Come!" wrote Louis Pasteur in 1871, "we will transform the world by our discoveries" (Moll, 1940). Pasteur's words seemed to portend the future of rural medicine as the Intermountain West entered the new century. Knowledge was being expanded in all fields, and medicine was no exception. Medical science had progressed impressively since the time that Sacajawea soothed her labor pains with powdered rattlesnake rattle, and increasing technological advances gave hope that life could not only be healthier but could last longer.

People began to realize that disease and infections were caused by living organisms and that cleanliness was a combatant against these phantom-like creatures they couldn't see. Other sound ideas about health care were accepted as fact in many of the more medically progressive urban areas, and some ideas began filtering into the isolated rural regions. But one discovery that had potential to transform the Intermountain Area's rural health care is often overlooked when medical milestones such as the germ theory and the X ray are discussed: Henry Ford's automobile, which changed rural medicine almost as much as Robert Lister's antiseptic surgery.

The Automobile Replaces the Horse

Pioneer doctors in the West knew that distance meant expediency . . . if a patient lived so far away that the doctor was unable to make repeat visits within a short period of time, the physicians often opted to amputate an arm or a leg rather than leave the patient in the care of inexperienced family or friends. Also, the long ride to outlying farms and ranches was tiring to the physician, resulting many times in poor or cursory treatment. But with the advent of the Model T, doctors were able to "commute" more easily and, certainly, more swiftly. One physician reported that his usual two-day journey to the hospital was cut to a day and a half after he traded his horse and buggy for an automobile!

But owning a car was no guarantee that the doctor would reach his patient without difficulty or even in the shortest possible time. As one rural physician of the early 1900s recalled half a century later (Howe, 1967):

> On one trip . . . a confinement case made during the month of January, I used four methods of transportation on the 21 mile trip. I first started out in my car with Dick Costello . . . as driver. After we had made about 12 miles, we got completely hung up in the snow. We started to shovel, and it seemed almost a hopeless job. . . . I left Dick . . . in charge of the car . . . and started walking with my heavy satchel toward the section house at Dumont. After I had walked about a mile, some boys came along with a team and sled. . . . I hopped into the sled and they very quickly took me to the section house. There the Burlington section boss got out his motor car, and after fixing a canopy to protect us from the cold wind, we proceeded 6 miles to Nahant.

By car, by walking in "32 degree below zero" weather, by riding in a sled pulled by horses, and by rail, the doctor finally got to his destination only to find "to my disgust . . . that it was a false alarm." His Hippocratic oath had prompted him to overcome the ordeals of the journey, but his anger at the family's disregard for his efforts brought this response:

> . . . I told those folks that so far as I was concerned, they would either bring the patient to the hospital or get another doctor, that I had made my last trip out there. They had hailed from Iowa and they proceeded to tell me how the Iowa doctors

> made these trips. I told them that they were now in South Dakota and that if they wanted my services, they would have to come in to the hospital. Strange to say, the baby was born about a week later, and they did get another doctor to go out. At that time, the weather was not so severe. The roads were plowed out and I understand that the trip was made without incident.

Not everyone was familiar with the automobile, and many who saw it for the first time were frightened by its peculiar appearance and the loud noises emanating from it. Horses belong in this category too, for a horse and car on the same road at the same time often resulted in panic for the animals and dismay for the driver. A relative of Edward Rich, a Salt Lake City physician, recalls an incident in the Salt Lake Valley (Rich, 1970):

> Horses of that day hated and feared the automobile, as if [they] realized it was sounding their own doom. On a trip to one of the settlements north of Ogden, Dr. Edward caught up with a couple of horses sauntering along the highway. Thinking to scare them a little to one side so he could pass, he tooted his horn. To his amazement, one of them blazed away and kicked one of the headlights out.

Dr. Rich's first car was an Oldsmobile with a single seat, a single cylinder, and chain drive, bought in 1903. After driving it but a short time, he purchased a second car, an "Elgin buckboard, with the motor over the rear axle." The doctor had to start the car by cranking it "from the rear [and then] sprint in a lively fashion to reach the seat and controls before the engine choked down or the car ran away." Although it was capable of a brisk fifteen miles an hour, the doctor found it too impractical and traded it for another Oldsmobile.

By 1911, two thousand inhabitants of Utah owned cars, but few traveled long distances because there were no road maps or even any signs along the road. Paved highways were not yet conceived, and the dirt and gravel roads that linked the nation disintegrated into mire during stormy seasons. According to Halliday (1957), the few courageous tourists who attempted to cross Utah condemned it as the "sand trap and mudhole of the West. . . . [I]t was not uncommon to stay stuck in a mudhole or hubcap deep in sand for a day or two until a farmer with a team of horses came by and hauled them out." And the inhabitants concurred.

The "Pathfinder." With the 1915 San Francisco Exposition approaching, Utah civic leaders decided that there was a bonanza of tourist dollars to be had if Utah's scenic attractions were publicized, the roads to them improved, and these roads charted. Thus in 1911, the Salt Lake *Tribune* hired sportswriter and auto enthusiast Bill Rishel, who had founded the nation's first auto club in 1903, to map Utah's auto routes. Rishel began his new assignment in an automobile labeled the "Pathfinder" (Halliday, 1957). Rishel's route information included warnings of "a bad mudhole" and "deep sand" on a trip to Wanship, Utah. Between Pocatello and St. Anthony (Idaho) was the "Ross Fork sand," of which Rishel said:

> . . . It is five miles long, but can be negotiated by deflating tires and taking your time. Indians with teams are stationed at both ends of this sand, anxious and willing to pull an automobile through for a small consideration. There are four especially bad spots. Extra passengers can help here by getting out and pushing.

Later, as manager of the Utah Automobile Association, Rishel published tour pamphlets that were similar but less sophisticated than those of today. Yet they contained maps, information on road conditions and tourist spots, and gave the kinds of information that a rural doctor would need to know about the roads he and his automobile would traverse. A 1931 pamphlet gave these facts ("Official Touring Guide," 1931):

> . . . Wendover to Gold Hill: Dirt road generally following the mud flat. Bad in wet weather. . . . Idaho Falls to Monida: U.S. Highway No. 91. Graveled highway. Main north and south road connecting Utah and Idaho with Montana points. Through a level farming and stock raising country. During winter months the Monida summit is closed with snow, and cars are shipped by rail from either Dubois or Spencer. . . . Nephi to Salina: About ten miles of graded dirt road, balance of route graveled highway. This is the shortest route between Nephi and Sevier valley points, optional highway through Salt Creek Canyon via Sanpete Valley. . . . In wet weather the direct route is likely to cause trouble with mud and in extremely dry weather it is liable to become dusty.

In Nevada, almost every doctor had a car instead of a horse by 1912. The percentage of car ownership was higher among physicians than the general public, but many people were now speaking of the auto as a positive influence on health care.

Cars Equal Health. If the automobile has no other virtue to recommend it, there is one that stands out – cars did not leave manure that had to be swept off the streets and stored in covered receptacles in a never-ending battle to keep shoes and skirt hems free of the filth. Besides, knowing that the doctor could arrive more quickly because of his automobile, some people's minds were set at rest. Many even believed that riding in a car was in itself healthful, claiming that the effort required to steer the vehicle helped to exercise muscles not used in walking. Others stated that it was an excellent treatment for tuberculosis, a cure for nervousness, or good for the digestion (Berger, 1973).

In a 1924 study by Mayers and Harrison, "The Distribution of Physicians in the United States," it was observed that the automobile had changed private medical practice, especially in the rural areas. For the first time, country doctors were facing competition and could no longer count on monopolizing a territory purely on the basis of proximity (Berger, 1973):

> With his professional conduct – more particularly what the laity deemed his professional mistakes and failures – his business affairs, and his personal life a subject of common knowledge and gossip in the village and roundabout, it was but part of the eternal constitution of things that a substantial portion of the residents of his territory should ordinarily be, if not actively dissatisfied with him, at least quite unenthusiastic about his merits, making use of his service only because no other physician was available.

When the rural inhabitants began buying automobiles, they found that they could consult better trained and equipped doctors in the nearby cities, and they often combined business or social trips to town with a visit to a physician. Partially as a result of this competition, rural doctors soon began a migration to the cities, producing a situation whereby medical care may have become less efficient in the farm or ranch communities than it had been before the automobile. Berger (1973) quotes from a 1923 *Ladies Home Journal:*

> The universality and convenience of the automobile have relegated the medical equine to the dodo class; the species is fast becoming extinct; but when roads are knee-deep in mud

or neck-deep in snow, we dwellers on countryside roads miss that noble nag and his trick of getting through somehow, sometime, when need calls.

Specialization Grows

The move toward specialization that began in the Intermountain Region in the early 1900s also took more physicians away from the rural areas and enticed them into the cities where they would have better access to highly technical instruments and facilities – and a more affluent clientele. As early as 1915, only 23 percent of all medical school graduates were general practitioners, while 36 percent were developing a specialty interest and 41 percent were entirely specialized (Stevens, 1971).

Billings, Montana, became the home of one of the area's early specialists when Dr. Carl Schulin, an ophthalmologist graduate of the University of Leipzig, Germany, and one of the founders of the Yellowstone Valley Medical Society, settled there in 1905.[1] It is the second member of the society, Dr. A. J. Movius, who is credited with spurring the move toward specialty care in the Billings area.

Dr. Movius, according to Edward Gibbs, M.D., medical director at the Billings Clinic, was a graduate of the University of Minnesota in 1904 and joined the local medical society in 1908. Movius was a close friend of Willard and Charles Mayo and a great admirer of the Mayo Clinic in Rochester, Minnesota. He believed that since Montana was so far removed from any major medical center, there was a superb opportunity to establish a clinic in Montana similar to the Mayo brothers' clinic, but on a lesser scale. In 1917 he hired an associate, Dr. J. H. Bridenbaugh who, after returning from military service in World War I, took graduate training in radiology and returned to Billings capable of doing both diagnostic and therapeutic radiology. Drs. Movius and Bridenbaugh were among the first twelve in the United States to purchase a 400 kilovolt X-ray unit which was at first in their office and later moved to one of the Billings hospitals. This was subsequently replaced by a cobalt unit.

In 1937, the clinic became known as the Billings Clinic. Dr. Gibbs says that Drs. Bridenbaugh and Movius gradually added to

---

[1]From correspondence between the authors and Dr. Paul Crellin, Billings, Montana, February 18, 1975.

their staff other physicians who had some specialty in specific fields of medicine; hence specialties in the Billings area flourished. "Because other physicians in Billings saw the value of specialty training exhibited by this group," said Dr. Gibbs, "they tended to seek other physicians with specialty training to provide competition for the Billings Clinic. Thus I would say the movement toward specialty care really got under way in the late 1930s."

Mrs. Ethel A. Taylor, administrative assistant at St. Vincent's Hospital in Billings, feels that another man who was partially responsible for the prodigious growth of medical specialties in Billings was Dr. Louis Allard, an orthopedist who came to Billings in 1922. "He did good work and really put us on the map as far as orthopedic medicine goes," she said. "He worked with polio patients and got them from as far away as the Dakotas and even Cheyenne, where the people could go just a hundred miles and be in Denver. His patients would go back to their homes and would spread by mouth the word about his success. Also, doctors heard about the good orthopedic work being done in Billings and this attracted more orthopedists. We still do a lot of orthopedic work because we have a crackerjack bunch of orthopedists."[2]

New medical instruments spurred the growth of many other Intermountain Area specialties, one of them being radiology. The first X-ray unit in Utah was bought in 1902, and while the identity of the buyer has been lost, a second machine, a huge static unit that took from five to ten minutes to make an exposure, was obtained later that year by a Salt Lake City physician, Dr. Augustus Behle (Wilson, 1973).

X Rays and Radiology. It was a layman, however, not a doctor, who became the first proficient radiologist in Utah. Louis Thody, trained in England for the electricians trade and who later moved to Utah as a convert of the LDS church, was hired in the early 1900s by the W. H. Groves LDS Hospital to be in charge of their electrical equipment, and as such, he was also in charge of their X-ray apparatus (Wilson, 1973).

> The equipment consisted of a ten-inch coil and electrolytic interrupter with a D'Arsonval high frequency resonator and two Leyden jars. There were eight or ten gas tubes of

---

[2]Telephone interview on January 14, 1974.

> various makes. The tube stand consisted of a wooden pole set in a metal base on casters and the tube was attached to the post with a sliding wooden clamp. The department was located in the basement adjoining the corridor leading to the laundry and garbage depository. The walls were painted black and the light source was a single chandelier and a small window at ground level. There was no dark room; the plates were sent to a downtown photographer for development. When an X-ray examination was required, one of the two interns at the hospital obtained the key to the department and, with the attending physician and patient, waited for the appearance of Mr. Thody. Then the plates were sent downtown for development. The procedure was totally unacceptable, so Mr. Thody established a "dark room," where processing was carried out in enamel trays with closely guarded secrets of chemical formula, developing time, etc. Ultimately, he used an electrical "rocking table" called a "titulator" which saved much time and effort on the part of the technician.

Despite problems (not the least of which was that at first the machine often failed to produce worthwhile results) and the fact that for some time an X-ray burn scare caused many of the new machines to remain idle (a university janitor had used his bare hands all day to demonstrate the wonders of fluoroscopy), doctors began to study the field and its instruments, and in the 1930s radiology became a board-certified specialty (Wilson, 1973).

At Last – Pure Food and Drug

The early 1900s brought not only automobiles and specialists to the Intermountain West, but also an increasing governmental and public awareness of health problems. This growing concern was felt all over the United States and was made official by Theodore Roosevelt when he signed the Pure Food and Drug Act in 1906. Sponsored by Senator Heyburn, its three main purposes were: (1) to eliminate all adulterations which might either be deleterious to health or tend to deceive, (2) to prevent all misbranding of food articles (that is, to compel every article to go upon the market under its true name and showing its true composition), and (3) to bring all of the diverse and antagonistic state legislation on the subject of foods to harmonize with the national law (McCumber, 1907).

Until this time, goods could be packaged and sold under almost any name, but worse than that, they didn't have to contain what they said they did. Even simple foods were easily adulterated; it was hoped that the Pure Food and Drug Act would, among other things, prevent spices and peppers from being mixed with "sand, sawdust, dirt, olive pits, nutshells, bark, bread, crackers, red dye, red sandalwood, rice, grain hulls, etc." ("The Pure Food Law," 1908).

It was also to do away with dangerous contents in drugs, whether obtained by a prescription or as a corner drugstore cure-all, for according to Heyburn, not less than 200,000 and perhaps 350,000 children lost their lives every year because of impure or misbranded drugs. While a breakdown detailing how many Intermountain Area children were affected is not available, it is almost certain that a large number were among the victims.

The turn of the century also brought an increasing trend toward urbanization. This, plus the greater awareness of health problems, made some sort of community control of sanitation and other health measures a necessity, since it was one thing when a family threw its garbage into the back yard after supper, but an entirely different matter when several hundred families did the same.

Sanitation – A New Awareness

Health matters had long been left to town councils, a practice which left rural areas without laws and gave the towns such ordinances as rural Morgantown's (West Virginia) 1849 ruling that no person be allowed to build a hog pen in the street or alley and that any hog running loose would be caught and sold by the city and the money kept as a fine.

A few local health boards had been established in the eastern states, but it was not until 1912 when a full-time health officer was appointed to promote the health of schoolchildren in Robeson County, North Carolina, that the first rural county health board was born. Since Robeson County had no town of more than 2,500 residents, its new organization could qualify as a rural one (Mott and Roemer, 1948).

Nevada Public Health. In the Intermountain Region, health boards and health legislation grew slowly. Nevada made a definite but feeble effort on behalf of public health in 1889, when county commissioners were authorized to establish and maintain county boards of health. The chief accomplishment from this was a public acknowledgment that health care was now becoming looked upon as more a communal idea, with needs of the people as a whole taking the place of frontier individualism.

But few actual advancements in Nevada's public health care were quickly seen. The Nevada State Board of Health was created in 1893, but was given limited funds, and the state legislature seemed to be more interested in livestock than in people. The sparsity of population kept many would-be epidemics from developing, making the need for such laws seem less necessary.

Nevada enacted some legislation in the first five years of this century, establishing a few county and city health boards, but no one was completely aware of any need for rural health supervision until 1905, when smallpox and malignant pneumonia broke out near the Goldfield mining district.

Many miners had come to Nevada during the winter; whether they found ore is unimportant. They did *not* find housing, sanitary provision, or pure water. The local saloon was the only warm building, and the miners slept on the floor in their wet clothes. Three to five deaths occurred each day, but county health officials either could not or would not take action to prevent these occurrences. State health officials visited the camp, were appalled at the conditions, but could do nothing to help (they, too, had no funds to spare). Finally, the state legislators and their constituents came to the realization that health officials must be given the means and the power to protect the rural community. Even then, the state board of health had to remain inactive until 1909 because, until that time, its members had not received more than $500 a year with which they could fund public health services.

In 1919, the legislature mandated that communicable diseases must be reported, thus allowing enforcement of quarantine. In 1925, it enacted a statute "forbidding the use of the common drinking cup and common towels on railroads and all public places; also, employers must provide separate lavatories for the sexes" (Walker, 1944). The germ theory had been accepted.

From 1937 to 1944, barbers, staffs of beauty salons, and food handlers came under the scrutiny of the public health department. Before this, men and women in advanced stages of syphillis or tuberculosis had been allowed to prepare food. M. R. Walker, an early-day Nevada physician, observed that if you wished to enjoy a meal, you should not sit where you could see into the kitchen.

Rural Health Departments. A seeming increase of public interest and additional state laws did not bring improved public health programs to the rural areas. As of December 31, 1934, only two states in the Intermountain West had rural communities, townships, or districts with full-time health officers ("Extent of Rural Health Service," 1935). Utah had two public health officers who served 30,383 rural residents (12.6 percent of the rural population) in one unit near Salt Lake City, the most populous and least medically deprived area of the state. Montana had four full-time health officers who served 35,139 rural residents (9.9 percent of Montana's rural residents). In Colorado, Idaho, Nevada, and Wyoming, rural inhabitants were without public health support, with 1,066,967 rural residents not receiving public health services. Large unserved areas of Montana and Utah brought the total to 1,602,744.

"During the last fifty years," Smillie (1947) says, "municipal health activities have advanced rapidly and effectively; meanwhile rural health administration remained stationary for generation after generation." Some state health departments attempted to meet rural needs by assigning specialists to visit areas at irregular intervals to aid and advise in matters such as disease control, or the establishment of maternal and infant health care centers. "Often the result is a sporadic 'campaign' of activity, which is of some educational value, but of little or no permanent benefit," Smillie says.

Health departments that did exist often lacked strength. They were usually headed by physicians who were overtaxed by their private practice and who had been given the formal title of "health officer" in order to conform with state laws or local ordinances.

Utah's Health Department. Dr. Samuel Beatty was the first appointed state health commissioner in Utah after it assumed statehood in 1896. In 1898, the Utah State Board of Health was created, with Beatty retained as its head but still on a part-time basis. According to Morrell (1956):

> The part-time basis of the appointment was to continue for many years, however, the law providing for a full-time health officer not being enacted until 1915. This was a serious

> handicap as the salary was small and the demands of the work sufficient to consume all of [the health officer's] time. The struggle to survive was a serious one, causing many anxious hours and much family concern.

Not only was the commissioner's salary small, in most cases he wasn't given enough funds to carry out even the minimum of plans. In 1932, those U.S. counties that did have a full-time health unit spent only 38 cents per capita, although leading public health officials claimed that the minimum amount should be $1.00 or $2.00.

Public health nurses tried to fill the gaps, but it was a difficult task. In 1931, the average ratio of public health nurses to people was a seemingly high 1:7,700; but in Utah the ratio was an even greater 1:13,400 (Utah State Planning Committee, 1936).

Public Health Nurse

Dorothy Lowman, a retired state director of public health nursing now living in Salt Lake City, was a public health nurse in Utah's Jordan School District from 1928 until 1934. She tells of some of the efforts there to improve health: "Out in Bingham we did a survey of how many children were malnourished – we inspected them and then instituted a program where the kids would line up and we'd give them the cod liver oil.

"We also, in Bingham, gave tonsilectomies en masse. Dr. Paul Richards was the mining company's physician out there, and we took all the kids that needed tonsilectomies and had a day or so in one of the settlement houses. We'd take out all the tonsils and take care of the kids until they were ready to go home. You'd get one ready while the doctor was taking another child's tonsils out, then take the second one in and the first one to the recovery room. Twenty or thirty children would be a hard day's work."[3]

But in many cases, when there were no functioning health departments, many of the rural people had never heard of such an agency, and others thought that they were for the poor only. The departments were often housed in dingy basement corners, and the populace felt that it could hardly be expected to provide guidance necessary to improve the health of the people. Good

---

[3]Interview, January 7, 1975.

leadership was a real problem because, until 1936, there was no training school west of the Mississippi for health officers or sanitarians.

Maternity and Infant Care – The Need Is Made Known

While legislators and others were toying with the idea of more government control for public health, one of the earliest demands that arose was for better infant and maternity care. Glover (1926) says:

> In practically all our ways we have outgrown pioneer conditions, but as far as child-bearing is concerned, for a considerable number of the mothers of the country, we might still be a country of disjointed and isolated colonies. Many women in the United States bear their children under the same conditions as the Pilgrim mothers. And there are inequalities of care in childbirth ranging from that of the skilled obstetrician combined with facilities of the modern hospital extending over nine months and costing as much as a thousand dollars or more, to the casual assistance of an untrained midwife limited to a few hours at the time of confinement and costing a few dollars, or perhaps as little as a quarter or a dozen eggs. For many women in isolated places, not even the ignorant midwife is there to stand by in the hour of crisis—no one but the husband or chance neighbor.

People seemed to think that childbirth was a natural function, that anyone who could easily get pregnant would surely have the baby with the same ease. Said Dr. Lottie G. Bigler (1920), a physician in Armour, South Dakota, in the early 1900s:

> I am reminded of a man who came to engage me to attend his wife who was near term. He said she hadn't been well for the whole nine months. I asked him why he hadn't consulted a doctor about her. He said he didn't think there was any need. He supposed they had to feel badly the nine months, she always had during her other pregnancies.

Good care and food for farm animals were provided, but the nutrition of children was often overlooked. The Intermountain Region was not alone in its problems, for in Kentucky, reveals *The Survey* ("For Blue Grass and Hill Babies," 1924),

> Demonstration conferences conducted at county fairs often revealed the fact that blue ribbon pigs and calves were given milk, but the most valuable animals of the farm, the children, were underweight and far from the blue ribbon class, because they drank coffee instead of milk. The good work of the county farm agent had set the right standards for hogs, but a standard for children was lacking.

In New York, according to *School and Society* ("The States and the Sheppard-Towner Act," 1923), a child hygiene appropriation was passed

> ...only after the Senate committee had been asked publicly and had to admit publicly that the Assembly had appropriated $125,000 each for two buildings at the state fair at Syracuse for the accommodation of swine. After which it was embarrassing to refuse the women's request for a corresponding amount to protect the health of babies.

An experimental appropriation for the health of mothers and infants and the first national recognition of the problem was the passage of the Federal Maternity and Infancy Act on November 23, 1921. Commonly called the Sheppard-Towner Act, it was to be planned and carried out individually by the states with the approval of a federal board of maternity and infant hygiene. The local administration was to be under the child hygiene of the child welfare division of the state; if there were neither of these, an agency would be designated by the state.

This act authorized an annual appropriation of $1,240,000 for a five-year period, of which not more than $50,000 could be expended by the Children's Bureau for administrative purposes and for the investigation of maternal and infant mortality. The remainder was to be divided among the states that accepted the act as follows: $5,000 unmatched to each state and an additional $5,000 to each state if matched; the remainder to be allotted among the states on the basis of population and granted if matched.

Forty-three states, including those of the Intermountain West, and Hawaii cooperated under the plan. Generally, the work fell into two categories: (1) educational stimulus toward better maternity care, and (2) the practical care and supervision of mothers through pre- and post-natal periods. Under the Sheppard-Towner Act's provisions, literature was distributed, correspondence courses held, and mothers educated to the needs of themselves and their children during pregnancy and infancy. During 1924–25, there were 9,669 prenatal conferences held, which were attended by approximately 75,000 women, with classes for midwives having an attendance of forty thousand. A total of 1,706 child health centers and 245 prenatal centers was established. Seven states obtained specially equipped cars that would facilitate examinations and demonstrations in rural areas.

Many physical problems were detected during these examinations, the most frequent being refractive errors in the eyes, nasopharyngeal growths and abnormalities, glandular enlargements or insufficiencies, orthopedic defects, cavities, and malnutrition. Children were referred to a doctor for corrective measures, or the problems were taken care of by staff doctors by some state programs. The rate of corrections was about 20 to 40 percent ("Working of the Federal Maternity and Infancy Act," 1925).

The Sheppard-Towner Act in Utah. When Sheppard-Towner funds became available in 1922, Utah State Health Commissioner Dr. Theodore Beatty asked the help of the women's organization of the Mormon church – the Relief Society – in carrying out Utah's plan. The Relief Society had sponsored training for nurses before hospital-trained nurses were available or even existent, and in 1920 had established courses in family welfare and actual field work, including the study of physical, mental, and public health. The women's work had affected thousands of homes and gave the Relief Society members a good background for carrying out the Sheppard-Towner directives (Morrell, 1956).

Utah soon had 194 health units throughout the state, and while Beatty got assistance from many agencies, in the rural areas the Relief Society was often the only organized group; thus these women shouldered much of the responsibility. According to Morrell:

> Under the law, no money could be spent from the appropriated funds for equipment . . . only for administration. The Relief Society came to the rescue and provided the necessary equipment, such as scales, linens, gowns, and many other items. They also provided the quarters for conducting the work, and the women to do the accessory work of conducting the clinics. This all proved to be a tremendous undertaking,

> but the work was done with dispatch. Local doctors were engaged for the examination under the direction of a doctor trained in the work of maternal and child health, and of public health as well. The doctors could now be paid for their services, although the compensation was limited. It was encouragement, however, and support was enthusiastically given.

Dr. Beatty later stated that, through the help of Sheppard-Towner, in Utah "there were 3,102 conferences held, 78,000 preschool children were examined, and 13,000 defects were reported."

The Sheppard-Towner Act continued until the appropriation period of five years had expired. Congress then extended the money for two more years but amended the bill so that funds would cease at the end of that time, thereby simultaneously extending and killing the Sheppard-Towner Act. But according to many, the main purpose of the act had been to stimulate the states toward better maternity and infant care, with hopes that the programs would continue after the bill's demise.

Medical Education – Intermountain Genesis

Another step toward better health care, which had fairly quick success once it got started, was the improvement of medical education. Through the first decade of the twentieth century, there was a paucity of medical education in the United States. Proprietary schools, whose main interest was the quick buck, flourished, and it was not unusual for a few doctors to obtain a college charter, steal some corpses, open a school in a barn, and make some easy money. There were no medical examining boards; a diploma was a license to practice. Schools gave their own examinations, but these were often brief and oral. At Harvard the rule was that any student who got the majority of votes from nine professors would be graduated, and most students succeeded even during a period when Harvard had only seven professors. By 1910, Missouri had produced 42 medical schools; New York, 43; Indiana, 27; and Tennessee, 17. In the city of Cincinnati alone, there were twenty medical schools (Flexner, 1910, 1973). The Intermountain Region attracted few proprietary schools, perhaps because of the sparse population or the early anti-doctor attitude of the Mormons.

A Utah Proprietary School? The earliest known medical school in the Intermountain Region was the Medical College of Utah at Morgan, founded in 1880 by Dr. Frederick S. Kohler. By 1883, according to Divett (1960), it no longer existed. But while it was in operation, with courses that lasted sixteen weeks, it graduated at least four persons. Whether it was a proprietary school is not known and, according to various records, is debatable.

Kohler, born in Pennsylvania in 1836, briefly attended Dartmouth but received his medical degree from the Eclectic Medical College of Pennsylvania in Philadelphia and the Medical College of Cincinnati. He claimed that he started the Morgan college because "there was both a practical and necessary call for it." His opinion was apparently shared by others, for 25 years later a medical college was established in Salt Lake City. But for reasons now lost to history, a Salt Lake City newspaper campaigned against Dr. Kohler's Medical College of Utah, causing its eventual demise.

It may have been because the little town of Morgan was strongly Mormon and Kohler was a Presbyterian, or perhaps it was because the newspaper's editors felt the medical school was not a good thing for the community that the school folded. Whatever the reason, the now defunct Salt Lake *Herald* began denouncing the medical school in the summer of 1882, saying in an editorial that the newspaper had investigated the school with the help of some Salt Lake City physicians and implying impropriety. In any event, a rebuttal was published by the school, but the paper retaliated with another editorial twice as scathing. Still more anti-medical school literature appeared and it was not too long before the town's confidence in the school was shattered. On August 26 the *Herald* published the following editorial (Divett, 1960):

> Dr. Kohler, the head and front of the pretended "Medical College of Utah" at Morgan City has left the country and gone to Denver. His departure was somewhat precipitate, occurring before the *Herald* had gotten through talking about him and his college. The doctor was entirely too tender-hearted. If he were engaged in no wrong doing he certainly ought not to have fled when he was mentioned in the paper, and if his college were regular and legitimate he shouldn't have been ashamed of having the world know all about it. There is no disgrace in being principal of a Medical College. When the *Herald* exposed the "Medical College of Utah" it

> had no intention or desire to drive Dr. Kohler out of the territory. Our only purpose was to warn the public, both in Utah and out, against an institution that showed crookedness on its face, and to prevent the sale of bogus diplomas of the Dr. Buchanan order. The doctor having admitted guilt by fleeing and letting his college collapse, we are not sorry that Morgan has lost its doctor and its medical institution that, according to some of their too enthusiastic dupes, were going to do so much to revolutionize the practice and price of medicine. Morgan may meet [*sic*] a doctor, but the county can afford to get along without a physician who engages in business that cannot be talked about.

Actually, however, Kohler remained a resident of Morgan until 1887, five years after the *Herald* campaign, training midwives instead of doctors. When he left Morgan, he moved to Nampa, Idaho, and became one of that town's leading citizens. Kohler died on January 1, 1908. The true answer as to whether the Medical College of Utah at Morgan was a "diploma mill" is still a mystery.

Medical Education in Colorado and Utah. Colorado's main experience with a diploma mill was the Denver Homeopathic College, organized in 1884 and reorganized several times thereafter, until it became extinct in 1909. Denver was also the home of the Gross Medical College which began as a proprietary school in 1883 when several doctors, denied entry into a recently formed medical school, decided to start a rival. Named after Samuel D. Gross, a distinguished surgeon, it grew and improved until by 1898 it had 71 students and was offering a four-year course of education (Jobe and Hills, 1958).

The school that had snubbed the Denver group was the Denver Medical College, founded in 1881 by the local medical association whose members had decided it was time Denver had a college of medicine. The first session began on November 5, taught by part-time professors who donated their time and often had to leave in the middle of a lecture if a patient from their private practice needed them. Clinics were held irregularly at the county hospital, and students were allowed to watch operations at nearby private hospitals.

Medical education at Denver Medical College, which took two years to complete, consisted of a six-month session each year. A high school diploma or equivalent was preferable, but without one, a prospective student was given an entrance examination which stressed writing, spelling, and composition.

The Denver college was not averse to good publicity to lure students to its school – its medical bulletins sounded like travel brochures:

> This city [Denver] is the Damascus of the West. Its beauty is the wonder of all who see it. Its intelligence is in proportion to its marvelous growth (pop. 75,000). Its churches are ably supplied and its schools are second to none in the country. Music and fine arts are widely cultivated. Colorado is the health resort of the Americas. Many thousands come here annually. The University offers to young people who cannot endure other climates, educational advantages equal to those of the best eastern colleges.

Considerable antagonism existed between these two Colorado medical schools. Officials of the Denver Medical College felt that there was no reason for the existence of Gross, and those at Gross in turn seemed to delight in taking verbal stabs at the Denver school through articles in the school's periodical, *The Gross Medical College Bulletin*. But by the turn of the century, mutual disrespect had faded, and the increasing costs of providing a good medical education had placed Gross in crucial financial straits. This, plus a growing belief among medical professionals that the number of schools should be decreased through abandonment or merger, caused the Denver and Gross colleges to join forces. In 1902 the Denver and Gross Medical College was born, with a four-year program that encompassed eight months of instruction and training each year. In the first year, there were 133 students and a teaching staff of 101.

A third medical college in Colorado was the University of Colorado School of Medicine in Boulder, started in 1883. The two members in its first class and those in several subsequent classes paid no tuition for their three years of instruction. The entrance stipulation was a high school diploma or its equivalent, or a passing score on an entrance examination. Many of the school's professors lived in Denver, commuting to Boulder once a week on the "Colorado Central," a local railroad.

Bad feelings arose between personnel at the Denver Medical College and those at the University of Colorado School of Medicine when, in 1893, professors of the Boulder school began teaching the last two years of the prescribed four-year course in Denver, where students could have access to better equipped hospitals. Many of the Denver staff were lured away from the Denver Medical College to the rapidly growing and improving facilities of the medical school in Boulder. In 1885, the course was lengthened from three years to four years. Tuition was $35 a year, special lecturers were engaged and, in 1896, a School of Dental Surgery was added.

Denver Medical College took legal action against its "rival" school in 1897 and the Colorado Supreme Court, declaring that it was illegal for the University of Colorado School of Medicine to hold classes in Denver, ordered its professors and students to retreat to Boulder. This was only a temporary setback, however, for a new forty-bed hospital was built in Boulder. The school also obtained use of the Colorado Sanatorium. Many of the Denver faculty resigned to join the Boulder school. By 1910, Boulder also had sixteen visiting physicians from Denver, making a total faculty of 44.

Permanent medical education in Utah, the only other state to have a major medical college in the Intermountain Region, began later than in Colorado. The University of Utah at Salt Lake City instituted its first two-year standard medical course in 1905, offering basic science courses. Although it was small, it apparently was a sound school for it withstood the criticism that was subsequently heaped upon all medical colleges – criticism that would change medical education in the United States and Canada.

For several years prior to 1891, colleges had been pressured to raise their standards of education and to give a more complete and higher level of training. In 1891, the National Confederation of State Medical Examiners and Licensing Board was established. Its members and those of the Association of American Medical Colleges urged medical schools to implement a four-year program with stiffer entrance examinations and stricter requirements. This reform movement met with resistance by many medical college officials who seemed to be more interested in student fees than student education. But eventually, official action made it mandatory that the medical schools either improve or close their doors.

The Flexner Report. In 1906, the Carnegie Foundation for the Advancement of Teaching took a positive step toward reform when it established a division for inquiring into the problems of higher education, including medicine. In 1908, the Carnegie Foundation and the American Medical Association decided to pool their efforts. Dr. Nathan P. Colwell, secretary of the AMA Council on Medical Education, and Abraham Flexner, an educator with the Carnegie Foundation, visited every medical school. Their findings were printed in 1910 as the book *Medical Education in the United States and Canada*, called the "Flexner Report." According to Stevens (1971), the report is an "extraordinary frank document, laying bare the skeletons and drawing the issues as Flexner and the council saw them." For the first time, medical schools were exposed by name, bringing public attention to many of the shocking classroom conditions and the often nearly complete lack of anything resembling a medical education.

The Denver and Gross Medical College fared better than many, such as the Maryland Medical College in Baltimore, which Flexner (1910, 1973) condemned as

> ... wretchedly dirty. Its so-called laboratories are the worst existing type: one neglected and filthy room is set aside for bacteriology, pathology, and histology; a few dirty test tubes stand around in pans and old cigar boxes. The chemical laboratory is perhaps equal to the teaching of elementary chemistry. The dissecting room is foul....

Yet Flexner was not overly impressed with the Denver and Gross school: "There is a total absence of scientific activity. The rooms are poorly kept. A few cases of books are found in the college office behind the counter." Hospital appointments, he said, were secured by "pull." He praised the dispensary building, calling it "new and exceedingly attractive." He was not so harsh on Boulder's school, for while Flexner felt that the clinical facilities were "inadequate" and the dispensary was "slight," he said, "The school is generally satisfactorily equipped as to undergraduate teaching in the medical sciences."

He recommended that the two schools merge, that all clinical facilities be moved to Denver, and that the state apportion more money to the medical college. Merger had been considered previously, but the Denver and Gross trustees had not been in favor of it. In the spring of 1910, the executive board of the Denver and Gross College of Medicine threatened the trustees that either the money must be supplied to improve Denver and Gross or the faculty would be unwilling to conduct the school as a second-rate institution. The board felt that the cost of improvement would be too expensive and withdrew their objections to merger, which was completed in January 1911 (Jobe and Hills, 1958).

The number of medical schools across the United States greatly decreased as a result of the Flexner Report. Many, like the Colorado schools, merged, but others closed their doors even before the investigation began so that they would not have to face Flexner's ruthless honesty. By 1920, there were only 85 medical colleges. With decreased quantity came a seemingly increase in quality. In 1905, only five schools required any college studies before medical school; by 1915, 85 demanded a minimum of one or two years, and by 1932, every recognized medical school and most of the state licensing boards required two or three years' work toward a college degree (Stevens, 1971).

The recently begun medical department at the University of Utah was one of the few that Flexner felt already offered a quality medical education: "Laboratories are adequately equipped for the routine instruction of small classes. . . . The spirit is excellent." The small school had only eighteen students and three full-time and three part-time professors.

Utah's Medical School Grows. By 1916, the Utah medical school was one of 67 in the United States (out of a total of 104) that had an "A" rating, according to new rating standards. In 1919 the School of Medicine, housed in the University's biology building, moved into a new brick building on the University of Utah campus that had been built as a dormitory for student officers in World War I. The war had ended before the building was completed, thus it was remodeled and became the home of the medical school for more than forty years.

Throughout the 1930s sentiment grew toward enlarging the program into a four-year course that granted an M.D. degree, since many of the graduates were finding it increasingly hard to transfer from the two-year course at the University of Utah to other schools of medicine. But there was also opposition to this idea. Some felt that Salt Lake City was not large enough to provide patients for a teaching hospital. Others thought the enlargement would be too expensive. Even the president of the university at that time wasn't sure it was a good idea. Despite opposition, in May of 1942 the Board of Regents approved the expansion, and students began using the Salt Lake County Hospital, several miles from campus, as a teaching facility. Under an accelerated program because of the World War II physician shortage, the first class graduated in 1944 (Salt Lake *Tribune*, 1975).

A faculty of outstanding quality was recruited, causing the school to be referred to as the "Johns Hopkins of the West," according to *Reflects*, a magazine sponsored by the University of Utah Hospital (1970). But the new four-year medical college was not without its problems. Space was at a premium; closets and toilets were converted into work space, classes were taught in stables, and an old G. I. latrine became a research laboratory. Still, says *Reflects*, "the medical profession was impressed by the vigor, the youthful facility, the dynamism and its rapid achievement of very high status among U.S. medical schools."

Selected References

Berger, Michael L. "The Influence of the Automobile on Rural Health Care, 1900–1929." *Journal of the History of Medicine and Allied Sciences* (October 1973), vol. 28, no. 4.

Bigler, Lottie D., M.D. "The Problems of the Expectant Mother in Rural Communities." *American Journal of Obstetrics and Gynecology* (December 1920), vol. 1, no. 3.

Divett, Robert T. "The Medical College of Utah at Morgan." *Bulletin of the Medical Library Association* (January 1960), vol. 48, no. 1.

"Extent of Rural Health Service in the United States, December 31, 1930–December 31, 1934." *Public Health Reports* (November 1, 1935), vol. 50, no. 44.

Flexner, Abraham. *Medical Education in the United States and Canada.* 1910. Reprinted, Buffalo, New York: The Heritage Press. 1973.

Foard, Fred T., M.D. "Need for Training Facilities for Public Health Personnel in the Western States." *American Journal of Public Health* (October 1936), vol. 26.

"For Blue Grass and Hill Babies." *The Survey* (September 15, 1924), vol. 52.

Glover, Katherine. "Making America Safe for Mothers." *Good Housekeeping* (May 1926), vol. 82, no. 98.

Halliday, Bob. "Utah's First Tourist." Salt Lake *Tribune*, Salt Lake City, August 4, 1957.

Howe, F. S., M.D. "Deadwood Doctor." *South Dakota Medicine* (February 1967).

Jobe, William E., M.D.; and Hills, David K., M.D. "The History of Medical Education in Colorado." *Rocky Mountain Medical Journal* (February 1958).

McCumber, P. J. "What the Pure Food Law Has Already Accomplished." *North American Review* (1907), vol. 184, no. 613.

Moll, Aristides A. "Half a Century of Medical and Public Health Progress." *Bulletin of the Pan American Union* (1940), vol. 74, nos. 1 through 12.

Morrell, Joseph R., M.D. *Utah's Health and You: A History of Utah's Public Health.* Salt Lake City: Deseret Book Company. 1956.

Mott, F. D.; and Roemer, M. I. *Rural Health and Medical Care.* New York: McGraw-Hill Book Company. 1948.

"Official Touring Guide of the Utah State Automobile Association Touring Bureau and Auto Club of Utah." Salt Lake City: Auto Tour Book Co. 1931.

"The Pure Food Bill." *The Outlook* (March 3, 1906).

"The Pure Food Law." *The Outlook* (August 8, 1908).

Rich, Junior Edward. *Happy Day.* Salt Lake City: Granite Publishing Co. 1970.

Roemer, Milton I.; and Faulkner, Barbara. "The Development of Public Health Services in a Rural County: 1838–1949." *Journal of the History of Medicine* (Winter 1951).

Rose, Blanche. "The History of Medicine in Utah." Salt Lake City: University of Utah. 1939. Master's thesis.

Salt Lake *Tribune*, Salt Lake City, Utah, August 4, 1967; January 26, 1975.

"The Sheppard-Towner Act before the Courts." *Congressional Digest* (March 1923), vol. 2, no. 2.

Smillie, Wilson G. *Public Health Administration in the United States.* New York: The Macmillan Company. 1947.

"The States and the Sheppard-Towner Act." *School and Society* (December 22, 1923).

Streeter, Carroll P. "Reorganizing Rural Health Facilities." *Public Health Nursing* (December 1935), vol. 27, no. 12.

Stevens, Rosemary. *American Medicine and the Public Interest.* New Haven, Connecticut: Yale University Press. 1971.

University of Utah Hospital. *Reflects* (July 1970), vol. 1, no. 5.

Utah State Planning Committee. "Health Conditions and Facilities in Utah." Salt Lake City: Utah State Planning Committee. 1936.

Walker, M. R. *Life's Review and Notes on the Development of Medicine in Nevada, from 1900–1944.* Reno: Private printing. 1944.

Wilson, Angus K. "How Radiology Became Established in Utah." *American Journal of Roentgenology Radium Therapy and Nuclear Medicine* (September 1973), vol. 119, no. 1.

"Working of the Federal Maternity and Infancy Act." *School and Society* (December 12, 1925), vol. 22, no. 572.

3

Hard Times — A Mighty Stimulus to Public Health

During the early 1900s, probably no other action had so profound an effect on medical education as the exposé of the Flexner Report. Since that time, however, many changes have seriously influenced medical education, such as the strong emphasis on research that arose after World War I and the more recent technological advances that helped to develop aerocosmic and atomic medicine. But in the area of public health, there is yet to be a stimulus comparable to the hard times of the Great Depression. The entire structure of health care changed with the sudden collapse of the U.S. economy on October 24, 1929.

Where before, people could afford to pay the small fees charged by doctors, clinics, and hospitals, now the majority was indigent — poorer than it had ever been in hard times. Unemployment rose to an unprecedented 25 percent by 1933. One man in four had no job, and the other three were forced to take drastic cuts in wages. When people had little money for food — to say nothing of money for clothing — they could not be expected to find a few dollars to pay for medical care. And those who had no money whatsoever, and were doomed to suffer most from malnutrition, were the saddest of the lot. Unemployment was more common than jobs, but ill health was the most common of all.

After Franklin D. Roosevelt's inauguration in January 1933, the President set about implementing a program which reflected his philosophy that for America to recuperate from its "disease of Depression," the federal government must play a larger, more persistent and more planned role in the economy. As part of his "New Deal," the Federal Emergency Relief Administration (FERA) was approved by Congress on May 12, 1933. Almost immediately, $500 million was made available for outright grants to the states for "relief." By the end of 1933, every state in the Union had an operating emergency relief organization that received money from FERA (Malmgren, 1965). Direct relief was then doled out by each state to its poor and indigent.

One of the major objectives of FERA was the establishment of "work-relief" jobs for employable workers on relief rolls, which were, according to Malmgren,

> ... based on the theory that needy workers may be jobless through no fault of their own; work relief is provided not primarily as a test of willingness to labor, but rather as a means of conserving the skills, work habits and morale of the able-bodied unemployed.... True work-relief undertakings, therefore, cannot be selected in haphazard fashion; emphasis is placed, rather, on securing a project which, when completed, will be of value to the community.

Utah's Emergency Relief Program

The FERA plan was instituted in Utah on March 31, 1934. When Utahns, rural and urban, became government employees, some of the projects they worked on not only helped them monetarily but also gave the state a chance to better the health of its inhabitants. For example, a hot lunch plan was instituted to "give employment to women while providing one hot dish at lunch time for undernourished children" (Malmgren, 1965). In Utah, 22 counties participated in this program; 95,331 children were served 1,551,254 meals, resulting in less absenteeism from school because of ill health and improved schoolwork for the children.

Public Health Nurses. Utah's emergency relief program hired unemployed nurses to set up a public health nursing network throughout the state. The program had an average of fifty graduate RNs, one or more from each county. The state was divided into five regions, with a public health nurse supervisor in each region. In addition, there was one state advisory nurse and one doctor who was employed as a medical relief adviser (Malgren, 1965).

One of the regional supervisors was Laverna Peterson, who in April 1934 began overseeing programs in the southern rural area of Wayne, Sevier, Piute, Garfield, Kane, Washington, Iron, and Beaver counties, with headquarters in Richfield, Sevier County. She worked there until 1936, when she was transferred to supervise eight northern Utah counties. During a January 7, 1975, interview, Ms. Peterson gave Piute County as an example of rural health conditions at that time when she stated: "We had done a survey of dental needs in the county, and they were tremendous. The people were very poor. They had just had a drought, and their diet was poor because of lack of variety – they had a lot of deer meat in season and some vegetables. More were selling their eggs than using them so they could get money for other things. We made arrangements with the school superintendent and had the children brought into Richfield. The dentist there would save that day and not take any patients from Sevier County, and the children would have their teeth worked on and then go play in the park.

"Sevier County itself was a county of eleven thousand people in scattered towns, and while they did have some doctors there, there were no ophthalmologists, and eye care was practically non-existent as far as having a good eye examination for a child. We were able to get the superintendent to okay using school buses on Sunday, and I talked with an ophthalmologist in Provo, quite a few miles away. He said he'd open his office on Sunday to fit glasses. We used the little medical relief money we had and put twenty children on the bus and took box lunches. The nurses would go along, and the children all took their turn having their eye examinations and having glasses fit. That was an unusual kind of arrangement for a rural area at that time."

She also related the case of a family in Garfield County: "One of the nurses asked me to go with her to see a family with impetigo. The whole family had it around their mouths and hands. Even the little baby had it, plus a sore bottom from not being kept clean and taken care of properly. To treat it, you had to go through a whole washing procedure with each child, and there wasn't even a wash basin in the whole house. Finally, we found a pan in the back yard that we could use as one. I showed the mother how to wash and treat the child, then made her do the same with the next one. The mother was somewhat retarded, so we had to keep repeating [the treatment]. The other nurse checked on them every day, and they all got well quite soon." According to Malmgren (1965):

> The benefits of the nursing program were many: more healthy babies and mothers due to proper nursing care; proper sanitation and supervision; women were taught personal hygiene and care of the sick in the home; communicable diseases were reduced in the schools; malnutrition and correctable defects were discovered in schoolchildren; and the program was of untold value to the scattered residents of rural counties where medical and nursing care are too difficult and too costly to obtain.

Mosquito Abatement. In early July 1934, the engineering department of Utah's Emergency Relief Administration prepared estimates and made applications for mosquito control projects in Box Elder, Cache, Davis, Salt Lake, Utah, and Weber counties. The mosquito in Utah, both as a pest and a disease carrier, was such a severe problem that abatement of this insect qualified as having the social and economic importance needed to qualify as a FERA recipient. (Earlier, in 1932, the Salt Lake Mosquito Abatement District had been formed, supported by general taxation funds, which laid a substantial foundation for the type of program that Utah's ERA could fund.) The 1934 program included open drainage ditches that would require "some rip-rap, drops, checks, culverts, bridges, and tile drains" (Malmgren, 1965). The tile was contributed by city, county, or state governments, or by property owners. Most culverts were donated by the sponsoring agencies. "Mosquito fish" were planted in breeding pools that could be drained. Many marshes were drained, thus eliminating breeding areas and adding water to the irrigation supply. Labor for these projects came from county relief rolls, with more than half of the timekeepers and foremen from the relief rolls also (Malmgren).

Community sanitation in Utah was sponsored by the Utah State Board of Health and operated under the supervision of the United States Public Health Service. Twenty Utah counties participated under the Utah ERA for "the elimination of unsanitary devices and conditions by the construction of sanitary privies in rural areas where sewers were impractical or not available" (Malmgren, 1965). Material for the sanitation projects was furnished by the sponsors, and the ERA of Utah furnished the labor. Altogether 2,172 sanitary privies were built, 276 sewer connections made, and 433 septic tanks installed. The Works Division projects under Utah's ERA were gradually closed out or transferred to the Works Progress Administration (WPA) established in 1935 by the President.

The Works Progress Administration

The WPA had been formed primarily to give locally sponsored, direct employment to persons who were able to work. It also was to coordinate the work of other federal agencies that were receiving federal emergency funds for construction. The health program of the WPA had four basic parts:

(1) Direct medical, dental, and nursing care for indigent people by employing jobless doctors, dentists, and nurses
(2) Projects designed to raise the health standards and eliminate unsanitary conditions, such as malaria control and drainage
(3) Establishment of curative facilities by building or improving hospitals, both general and special
(4) Projects designed to assist in medical research and the development of special types of therapy and of medical techniques

The WPA began in Utah on July 1, 1935, when the regional conference of the WPA met in Salt Lake City to organize the eleven western states into a functioning unit of the program. The Utah State Board of Health sponsored the first WPA project in Utah, which started on September 12, 1935, and which was similar to one of the Utah ERA rural endeavors: building privies. Known as the Community Sanitation Program, its workers, by 1938, had installed 17,716 sanitary privies, more than half the outdoor sanitation facilities of the entire state. These privies were secured to a slab of concrete that had been poured directly on the ground, surrounding the pit. They cost between $18 and $30, a sum that property owners paid, but the work was done by WPA employees. According to the state board of health, these outdoor toilets brought a reduction in cases of filth-caused contagious diseases.

Until the advent of the WPA, many rural and semi-rural areas had no central culinary water system. Wells or flowing creeks supplied the water for cooking, bathing, cleaning, and drinking. Seldon Anderson, mayor of Oak City, a tiny hamlet in Sevier County, said of the WPA, "One of the biggest assets to our city was the project of our culinary water system, wherein 100 percent of the residents receive direct benefit. In the years gone by, it was always the family at the head of the ditch that had the best water for culinary purposes" (Malmgren, 1965).

Many other WPA projects doubtless affected the Intermountain Region, although the majority was likely carried out in the more populated regions. Yet the rural inhabitants also benefited from these projects, including establishment of medical clinics (giving jobs to professionals and health care to the needy), drainage projects to lessen the irritating mosquito, and hospital construction and improvements. Two other aspects of WPA should be discussed briefly here, one in Utah and the other outside the state but having an effect on its population.

Adult Education. In November 1935, the WPA began offering adult education courses, one of which was in home hygiene and the care of the sick. Sponsored by the Utah chapter of the American Red Cross, the course was conducted in the Utah cities of Provo, Spanish Fork, Payson, and Pleasant Grove. In all, 155 persons enrolled in these courses, with 121 completing and receiving certificates. Although this is but one of the various topics taught in adult education, it was vital to the health needs of the state. Other adult education courses were conducted in more than a hundred communities of almost every county of the state (Malmgren, 1965).

Whooping Cough. One program that affected the residents of the Intermountain Region was based outside the area. The WPA granted funds to the Michigan State Department of Health to isolate the whooping cough germ and develop a serum for the child-killing disease. In Utah, which had an especially high rate of deaths due to whooping cough, the case rate per hundred thousand population in 1935 was 1,254, compared to 71 in Colorado and 33 in Idaho. A study of sixteen states (Utah State Planning Committee, 1936) showed that Utah had the highest morbidity rate, and generally a higher mortality rate, from whooping cough during the years from 1920 to 1935 than any of the others. It was also discovered that whooping cough was one of several communicable diseases having a combined death rate 34 percent higher in rural areas than in urban places. As a result of the Michigan efforts, health officials throughout the United States were able to bring the disease under control, with cases of whooping cough nowadays rarely causing death in children and infants, unless complicated by other health problems.

The Public Works Administration

Other Depression-era government relief projects came under the auspices of another Roosevelt agency, the Public Works Administration, established in 1933. Its effect on the Intermountain West was maximal, for by 1940 it had provided 121,760 hospital beds at a cost of $377,644,883 – the equivalent of five years' growth under normal conditions.

Of all PWA work at the state level, 11 percent was for construction of sewer systems. Approximately 67 percent of all new sewage treatment plants built from 1933 to 1940 were PWA projects (Carmody, 1940).

The Civil Works Administration

Established November 9, 1933, the Civil Works Administration spread its funds rapidly – in Utah, work under the CWA began on November 19 of that year. The agency was set up to provide jobs both for those on the relief rolls and those who, for various reasons, were not (Rasmusson, 1942). Two of its many projects in Utah include the construction of the Carbon County Hospital in Price and improvements to the Salt Lake County Hospital. Through the CWA, irrigation systems were improved in four Utah communities and drainage was bettered in Newton, Hyrum, Roosevelt, and Salt Lake City. Sewer systems were built in Brigham City and Cedar City and improved in Millard, Kaysville, and Delta. The program also directed nursing projects in six counties and culinary water supply improvements in 35 towns.

The Civilian Conservation Corps

Although the New Deal programs discussed thus far were profoundly beneficial to the health and economic recovery of the Intermountain Region, it was the Civilian Conservation Corps that involved the young people of the area, giving them job opportunities when there were none to be had in the larger market. Started in Utah in the summer of 1933, by June 1938, a total of 15,912 young men had participated in the program. They received $30 a month as wages, but they were also housed, clothed, fed, and given medical attention.

The operation of the CCC program was fairly extensive in Utah because of the many national parks within the state's boundaries, and also because of the extent of public domain lands controlled under provisions of the federal Grazing Act. Six of Utah's 26 CCC camps in 1938 were populated entirely by young men from Utah, all between the ages of seventeen and 23, unmarried and unemployed, plus many Utah men were employed as non-enrolled personnel, such as work project assistants.

The state benefited by many of their health-oriented projects— the clearing of irrigation channels, improvement of water supply systems, and rodent control (which included 843,244 acres of pest-ridden sites throughout the state) (State of Utah, 1939). Although the Civilian Conservation Corps, with its companion agencies discussed earlier, was abolished when the U.S. Supreme Court declared these agencies unconstitutional, it helped to enrich the lives of the citizens of the Intermountain West, not only by providing jobs for the unemployed, but by upgrading medical facilities and health care throughout the West.

Construction of Hoover (Boulder) Dam

A project that was to have singular impact on the health as well as the economy of the Intermountain Region was construction of the Hoover Dam near Boulder, Nevada. Called Boulder Dam when it was constructed (1931 to 1936), it later was renamed for President Herbert Hoover and called Hoover Dam.

The Industrial Commission at Carson City and the Bureau of Reclamation required the contractor – Six Companies, Inc. – to set up a full-time health department to care for the health and safety of the workers and to build a permanent hospital at the site (Walker, 1944). The hospital, at the cost of $90,000, boasted sixty beds and all of the standard equipment of the era: X-ray and fluoroscopic units, diathermy, infra-red and mercury quartz lamps, facilities for complete blood and urine work, a pharmacy, and five staff doctors.

The health care requirements proved justifiable, for during the forty million man-hours of work, more than 5,200 reportable industrial accidents occurred, from four to fourteen of these a day requiring a doctor's care. One to seven men entered the hospital each day. There were 97 industrial deaths and 112 nonindustrial deaths while the dam was being constructed.

Heat Prostration. Among the health problems that accompanied building the Hoover Dam were heat prostration and exhaustion, with 150 cases and seventeen deaths occurring in the summer of 1931. Concerned over the high number of cases, the Bureau of Reclamation and the contractors established a laboratory in Boulder City where experiments were performed not only on men but also on dogs. When it was found that workers were losing salts as well as fluids in the hot Nevada sun, they were encouraged to increase their salt intake, and extra salt was added to the food, when practical, at the commissary. Dispensers of five to ten grains of sodium chloride were placed in conspicuous places round the construction site, and men were urged to drink large amounts of water. Newcomers to the work site were placed on jobs that were not in direct sunlight until they became acclimated to the heat.

Other Health Precautions. To help prevent communicable diseases, all those who sold, handled, or served food were regularly inspected. No food handlers were hired who had a history of having been in or near northern Illinois within a six-month period prior to coming to Nevada to work on the dam, for a severe outbreak of amoebiasis occurred there in 1933. As a result of this precaution, the camp was free of the disease.

Meticulous care was taken in handling the milk, and producing its by-products, from the camp's 125 tuberculin-tested cows. The only known case of milk-borne infection was traced to butter brought in from Idaho. Protective equipment – helmets, belts, goggles – was mandatory at all times for men whose jobs were in a hazardous area. And first aid classes were held once a week for the employees, with instructors on first aid being placed throughout the project during working hours.

A Final Word

Throughout the Intermountain States, steps were being taken toward economic recovery, and many of these steps significantly improved people's health during those troubled times. But it was not until the government set up programs specifically aimed at health care that people were able also to begin a recovery from the medical problems inflicted upon them by the poverty of the Great Depression.

Selected References

Carmody, John M. "The Federal Works Agency and Public Health." *American Journal of Public Health* (August 1940), vol. 30.

Malmgren, Larry H. "The History of the WPA in Utah." Logan: Utah State University, 1965. Master's thesis.

Rasmusson, A. Vernon, "The Government Work Relief Project in Utah, 1932–40." Salt Lake City: University of Utah. 1942. Master's thesis.

Utah State. "First Biennial Report of the State Department of Public Welfare." Salt Lake City: *Utah State Public Documents*, vol. 3, no. 25. 1939.

———— Planning Committee. "Health Conditions and Facilities in Utah." Salt Lake City: Utah State Planning Committee. 1936.

Walker, M. R. *A Life's Review and Notes on the Development of Medicine in Nevada.* Private printing. 1944.

"The WPA and Public Health." *American Federationist* (June 1938), vol. 45, no. 6.

4

The Farm Security Administration Tries Medical Cooperatives

Even though the government programs brought jobs and money to many, major portions of the U.S. citizens were still facing hard times, especially the farmers. By 1935, three million farm families throughout the nation were experiencing not only the agricultural market's slump following World War I, but also the reaction to the collapse of the stock market, with its far-reaching worldwide Depression. The drought of 1934, which had been building since 1933, added to their woes, causing many of them to give up their farms and try to find employment in the cities.

In the Intermountain West, farmers were no different. Farm prices were at an all-time low, and farmers were subsisting on whatever they could grow on their lands. Some piled their produce into automobiles or wagons and took them to nearby towns and cities in an effort to get cash for other necessities.

In Utah, the farmers' plight was intensified, for many farmers' individual holdings were in different spots throughout the valleys. A man might own an acre or so near his home and another parcel of land a few miles away or, in some instances, several small acreages in several widely separated areas. This method of farming, more costly than if the land were all in one place, had already placed added burden on the Utah farmer because he could not compete with the large farms of the Midwest that used machinery to harvest the crops. When the Depression came, there were thirty thousand farmers in the state, each with his own farm acreage, and many were forced to sell their land and look elsewhere for employment, some even going to another state. Those who stayed weathered the "dust bowl" era of the mid-1930s, knowing that theirs was a smaller loss than that of the Midwest farmers.

Governor Henry Blood's "State of the State" message to the people of Utah in 1935 portrayed the seriousness of the situation (Stout, 1971):

> No report of the condition of the state during the past biennium would be complete without mention being made of the devastating drought that swept over Utah in 1934. No county in the state escaped its ravages. Mountain, valley, and plain were all involved. Destruction of livestock feed on both summer and winter ranges was an outstanding aspect of this disaster. Cash crops usually relied upon by farmers to provide funds for current needs and for payment of taxes were reduced in volume and in some localities were completely lost.

The precipitation in 1933 was actually less than that in 1934, but the continuing lack of rainfall, plus higher temperatures in 1934, brought on the most intense drought that Utah residents had ever witnessed. According to E. Arlo Richardson,[1] Utah State Climatologist at Utah State University in Logan, the Palmer Drought Index is the standard method of measuring drought intensity, with a minus 4 (–4) classified as "severe drought." From March to October 1934, the Palmer index in Utah's North Central Division, which includes Cache Valley and the "Wasatch Front,"[2] was:

Month	*Index*	*Month*	*Index*
March	–5.77	July	–9.06
April	–7.06	August	–8.61
May	–8.27	September	–7.74
June	–8.83	October	–7.26

Record-breaking drought such as that suffered by Utahns in 1934 has not been recorded since then.

---

[1]Telephone interview, July 16, 1975.

[2]A term used by Utahns denoting the area along the west face of the Wasatch Mountains, extending from Brigham City in the north to Provo and beyond in the south.

The Farm Security Administration

Roosevelt's Administration recognized the farmers' plight and took steps to help these families. Out of the FERA grew a rural rehabilitation plan, the Resettlement Administration, later known as the Farm Security Administration. It made low-interest loans to farmers, enabling them to purchase seed, farm animals, equipment, buildings, more land, and other needs. As self-sufficiency increased, the farmers were able to pay off the loans after selling their crops and stock.

Some farmers, however, were unable to repay their loans. The agency investigated (two years after the loans were made) and found that nearly half of the farmers who defaulted were in poor health. In truth, their farm animals were in better health than the farmers for, if a mule or cow got sick, FSA funds were available to pay for a veterinarian's help. But if the farmer himself was in ill health and asked his FSA supervisor for assistance, he often found that doctors willing to help were out on house calls, and those near by refused when they learned that there was no remuneration for their services.

Questionnaires sent to FSA families in Texas and Oklahoma, reported in a 1942 issue of *Public Health Nursing* (Goding, 1942), showed that of 43,000 replies, there had been sixteen thousand illnesses, less than half of which were treated by a physician. In addition, one out of every three children had been born without a doctor's help. Strangely, the doctors who treated these seemingly seldom treated people were left with a half-million dollars of unpaid medical bills (Goding, 1942).

Most poor families avoided the doctor if possible, but if a family member's cold turned to pneumonia, every effort was made to effect a cure, including a visit from the doctor (or to the doctor) and worrying about the bills later. Loans from FSA were defaulted as farmers sold their FSA-bought pigs, cattle, and equipment to pay for medical bills. When the money ran out, they were faced with one of two choices — let the doctor fees go unpaid or die because of lack of medical attention.

It became apparent that many successful farmers were not in this circumstance because they were lazy, as some thought, but because they were ill. County supervisors traced difficulties to acute illnesses, abscessed teeth, hernias, and other ailments. Dr.

R. C. Williams, a county doctor who was aware of the medical care problems of both patients and doctors, says (1940):

> Aside from the wanton waste of human life and curtailment of borrowers' usefulness to themselves, some kind of medical care program was plainly indicated to the Farm Security Administration from a purely economic point of view.

The result was that funds for medical care – perhaps $20 or $30 a year – were included in FSA loans. But it was difficult to predict how much money, if any, a family might need. The only feasible approach seemed to be a group plan in which each participating FSA family would pay a low annual fee into a local fund, placing family members under the care of one or more physicians who had agreed to treat them. In 1936, the U.S. Public Health Service loaned Dr. Williams to the FSA to help devise a suitable group health insurance plan. His plan was based on four principles (U.S. Congress, 1943): (1) free choice of physicians, (2) group payment, (3) family contributions based on average incomes, and (4) voluntary participation.

FSA in the Intermountain West

The states' official experiences with FSA medical programs are difficult to document because five years after any corporation is abandoned, the records are destroyed, according to Dennis Winter,[3] chief of Community Programs, Farmers Home Administration, Salt Lake City. In addition, county records are held only until loans are repaid, usually three to seven years, says Teresa Harmsten,[4] County Clerk, Roosevelt (Duchesne County), Utah.

However, it is known that in the Intermountain Region as of June 30, 1943, approximately the time that the FSA plans were at their height throughout the country, there were eighteen counties covered by FSA medical programs in Colorado, giving medical service to 1,233 families and 5,262 people (U.S. Congress, 1943). In Idaho, 21 counties were participating, with 792 families and 4,013 people receiving medical service. Montana plans included

---

[3]Telephone interview, December 5, 1974.

[4]Telephone interview, December 5, 1974.

37 counties, 2,121 families, and 10,352 people; Utah, five counties, 658 families, and 3,440 people; and Wyoming, eleven counties, 520 families, and 2,566 people. Because of Nevada's small number of FSA borrowers, that state did not become involved in the medical aspect of FSA.

Before a plan was set up, an agreement was reached with the state medical society, and the approval of the local medical society which supervised the medical aspects, was obtained. Any or all doctors in the area could participate if they desired, with patients having free choice in selecting one of these physicians.

Annual dues for the family were paid in advance, the money being put into a common fund controlled by a bonded treasurer or trustee who made the monthly payments to the physicians, usually based on a fee-for-service plan (Mott and Roemer, 1948). Some plans used the capitation (per capita) fee method, in which each FSA doctor received a flat fee for each family under his or her care, irrespective of the amount of service rendered. Others put their doctors on salary, with a per-hour fee in some of the dental plans arranged later in the program. Payment in kind, in which the farmer paid part of his bill in cash and part in farm produce annually to the local hospital, was accepted by some cooperatives.

Dues were based on average income of FSA borrowers in each plan and were according to services available or, sometimes, size of family. If a borrower could not meet the annual initial payment, which during research was found to range from $12 to $72, but desired to join, the FSA increased the amount of the original loan. No FSA borrower was forced into the medical plan. It was presented to the farmer and the choice was his; but in many cases, joining was an economical necessity.

Fee for Service. In a typical FSA program, a fee-for-services plan, the doctors presented bills at the end of the month. These were reviewed by a committee of local physicians who checked for improprieties, such as too many calls being made for the diagnosis, and fees that were approved were paid from the common fund which was divided into twelve monthly allotments. If there was money enough, bills were paid in full; otherwise, they were paid on a pro rata basis. Money left over was held until the end of the year, when it was applied to bills outstanding. Any funds remaining after that were used to supplement the next year's funds. Medical benefits usually covered in FSA plans included (Williams, 1940):

> . . . (a) ordinary medical care, including examination, diagnosis, and treatment in the home of the family or office of the physician; (b) emergency surgery necessary to save the life or limb of the individual as determined by the physician in charge of the case; (c) emergency hospitialization believed necessary and recommended by the attending physician; (d) obstetrical care, including prenatal, delivery, and postnatal care services; (e) ordinary drugs dispensed or prescribed by the attending physician; and (f) in some areas, dentistry prescribed by the attending physician and believed necessary to relieve acute symptomatic disease or to relieve pain.

Some of the poorer areas of the nation, of course, received fewer services, for the farmers there could not afford the high fees for medical and dental care; but nearly all programs provided at least general practitioner services.

One such program, which began in the late 1930s and extended into the early 1940s, was in southeastern Idaho. Although others were subsequently formed, this was perhaps the first in the state, according to Dr. H. L. Schiess,[5] a general practitioner in Shelley, Idaho, from 1935 to 1945, and now a surgeon in Seattle.

Idaho and the FSA. Schiess says that there was "only one health program in Idaho for the rural poor and that was in southeastern Idaho where the population was almost entirely rural. The LDS church helped some people pay their bills, and industries had medical programs, but there was only one program for the rural people that I am sure of."

He recalls that the FSA program was not run by the prepaid method used by most states. "The government paid for it entirely. Prices were set at about one-third the cost, and the government would pay the doctors for their work. . . . It was a very minimum service program. We gave physical examinations, did mostly office calls and general aches and pains. I did do some appendectomies, hysterectomies, and c-sections, and I took out tonsils."

Before the FSA started this program, says Schiess, many of the doctors saw few of their bills paid by the poor families; thus they donated their services, having to defray their own expenses. "We had office girls to pay and medication to buy, and that all came out of our own pockets. We would have had nothing at all if the gov-

[5]Telephone interview, January 6, 1975.

ernment had not paid the bills. Many of the doctors were afraid of it [the FSA], especially the older ones. They were afraid the government would take over medicine and it would become socialized, but I was young and couldn't see it that way."

At the time of this program, it was not medical care that people lacked, says Schiess, but rather medical science. "There were no antibiotics, so many people were hospitalized for things that today we would treat with antibiotics. People died of pneumonia, and there were small pox epidemics. Besides that, many people weren't convinced that vaccination was the right thing to do, and there were no laws [regarding] vaccination as there are now. But health care in Idaho was not poor; the doctors took care of the people. . . . I would never turn anyone away who came to me, and there were enough doctors to go around. There was just that lack of knowledge."

In a letter dated February 9, 1942, Schiess and Dr. Edwin Cutler, also of Shelley, wrote to a House committee on agriculture, which was investigating the activities of FSA (U.S. Congress, 1943):

> . . . Living in a small community, a physician comes in very close contact with his patients, both from a moral and financial standpoint. We feel that a great number of our patients who owe us money are those who have had misfortunes occur to them. Consequently, when they become so far in debt, they sort of give up, as they see no reason to pay one bill and let the others go. This gives them a "don't care" attitude. . . . We do think that the Farm Security Administration is doing a marvelous work in rehabilitating unfortunate individuals who really do want to get ahead and keep their self-respect and credit. Therefore, we feel that there is a great future in this work and that the organization should continue to function.

The FSA in Utah. Sources from different years show that there were several medical cooperatives in Utah, beginning in 1940. They came into being and then died out, but their documentation is preserved in publications from that era. In 1940, San Juan, Wayne, Grand, and Box Elder counties had group programs (Hellman, 1940). In 1943, five counties (U.S. Congress, 1943) were listed as participating in farm medical cooperatives; while in 1946, there were eight plans in thirteen counties, according to Ziegler *et al.* (1947). Interviews and research reveal that programs did indeed exist in Uintah, Duchesne, Utah, Sanpete, and Sevier counties, the last two being dental programs. Dental programs for Cache, Rich, Duchesne, and Uintah counties got at least as far as the planning stage, and possibly farther.

"It seems like we covered an awful lot of territory," says D. Ivo Eames,[6] past state director of the Farm Security Administration, now retired and living in Bountiful, Utah. "We were all thrilled to get a medical service into those areas. . . . For many years while I was in government, all they had in Wayne County was a nurse in Loa. It was kind of a joke about how many babies were delivered in the car – I don't think they had an ambulance – on the fifty-mile trip to the hospital in Salina."

In 1940, two thousand people lived in Wayne County, "a county with only one telephone line to Loa, the county seat, and in other ways semi-isolated from other parts of the state" (Salt Lake *Tribune*, 1943). There were 250 families living there, and thirteen hundred people joined the medical plan when it was started.

"We hired a doctor from Chicago for Wayne County and kept him there for more than two years," recalls Eames. "We got him an office in Loa, and the people came in as they needed to for sickness, and he made house calls. It cost twenty-five dollars per family per year, and it worked out quite well. . . . I remember when that doctor was to get his first check. It was a few days late, and he had really given up a lot to come to Loa – he'd transferred his whole family and everything he had out there. Anyway, his check was late and he sent me this terrible letter and really scorched me. He told me all these terrible things he was going to do.

"When I got the letter I really didn't understand what it was all about, so I went right out there and found out he was upset about his check. The farmers in the co-op were to pay him and it turned out that they took things kind of easy – they didn't figure a day or even a week or two would matter; they knew they'd pay him. But he didn't look at it like that. We got his check written out for him that day. It worked out alright, but for a few hours there was a lot of worry."

But by 1943, the Wayne County situation was not so good. The doctor from Chicago had left and had been replaced by Dr. S. W. Smith who also wanted to leave when his contract was up

[6]Telephone interviews, January 14 and 17, 1975.

at the end of January. Fred Brown, president of the Wayne County Medical Association, warned (Salt Lake *Tribune*, 1943):

> Being without the services of a resident physician would be bad, particularly at this time, due to the gasoline and rubber shortage, a lack of communications, the mountain road to Sevier County being closed occasionally by heavy snow and wind, and the shortage of doctors in Sevier County.

Residents of Wayne County were from fifty to 125 miles from Salina and Richfield, where the nearest doctors lived and practiced.

Dr. Smith eventually left, and Wayne County could find no doctor to replace him. "When Smith left, the program died in Wayne County," says Eames. "But while it was going, if kids got hurt, broke an arm or something, they got attention right quick. I'm sure a lot of people had their lives extended because of the program."

Another Utah medical plan was in Uintah County from 1941 to 1943. When Freda Davis, a home supervisor for the FSA in Vernal at that time, was asked if she remembered it, she responded quickly, "You bet! We [the FSA] negotiated it ourselves with the doctors, and it cost each family thirty dollars, prepaid, per year to join. All FSA borrowers were eligible, and the government loaned them the money. It was a marvelous program, and it covered everything. It paid maternity care – a high percentage of the borrowers had babies while on the program, and it gave them pre- and postnatal care. Broken legs, office calls, and surgery were taken care of for everyone in the family. And a lot of them had very large families."[7]

As an FSA home agent, Ms. Davis helped in other health and hygiene matters, such as advising wives on nutrition problems, or helping to make mattresses out of cotton. "I remember we made so many [mattresses] and the cotton was so dirty that I had a bad cough for a long time. Also, the FSA distributed sanitary privies – we called them "Roosevelt memorials" – and helped to build cisterns so the people could chlorinate their water. . . . The medical program was optional, but a lot of people signed up. Our case load was about two hundred families back then, so I imagine about two hundred families were involved.

---

[7]Telephone interview, January 6, 1975.

"They were all thrilled by it [the FSA medical program]. But the doctors gave too much service for what they got. We sold it to them on the idea that they would get money from some people whom they usually treated for free, and that if each family paid thirty dollars, those who didn't get medical service would make up for the cost of those who got more than thirty dollars' worth. The trouble was – everybody got more than thirty dollars' worth. The doctors got dissatisfied and wouldn't join up and honor the program anymore."

One family who received considerable use from its FSA medical plan membership was that of Eldon Billings of Vernal. Now retired from his machinery business but still farming because "it's in my blood," Billings[8] recalls that in 1941 he had three children, thus there were five family members on the program. "I started to farm that year. I got an FSA loan of five hundred dollars and bought five shorthorn cows and quite a lot of equipment. The cows cost fifty to sixty dollars apiece, and my mowing machine was a hundred and seventy-five dollars. I'd just started farming when I got an attack of appendicitis. . . [and was hospitalized] for three weeks. . . . I remember it happened in June, because I was just getting ready to put my hay up. While I was gone, my neighbors put up fifty tons of hay for me."

Billings paid $30 for his entire stay in the hospital that year. Another year, it paid for his wife's appendix operation and for his oldest daughter's broken arm. "I've had so darn many accidents that it's hard to remember any one in particular," he added. "Once, though, I was working the road with a four-horse fresno – that's a scraper and was the only way we had to get the dirt then, as we didn't have bulldozers. Well, I got in an accident with that, and I broke a rib, and it bruised me up.

"Another time, when one of the boys was five or six or seven, the kids were blowing cottonwood buds through willow tubes. In the spring, if you take a willow twig and beat the wood, you can slip the inside out of the bark; and I made a bunch of these tubes for them to play with. They were shooting them at one another. My boy hee-hawed when he hit another boy in the eye and he [the Billings boy] sucked in and [inhaled] a bud. It went down into his lung and swelled up like a tadpole, I had to take him to

---

[8]Telephone interview, January 9, 1975.

[a hospital] in Salt Lake City. It cost three hundred dollars, and the FSA paid the whole thing."

What would Billings have done without the FSA medical plan? "Well, the doctors would have had to wait a while for their money until I made it." At that time, Billings was earning approximately $50 a month.

Dental Cooperatives

By the time dental cooperatives were instituted in 1939, providing dental care to borrower families had become a staggering problem for the FSA. Dental disease, basically caused by neglect, was almost universal among low-income farm families. Although annual dental checkups are the most effective preventive of dental problems, these people had not received even cursory care and the accumulation of dental defects was immense. According to the FSA report (U.S. Senate, 1943), a 1939–40 survey of 2,480 FSA borrower families (11,479 people) across the United States revealed that the most prevalent defect was dental cavities. Of all those examined, the survey showed, 69 percent had decayed teeth, and 85 percent of white persons between the ages of fifteen and thirty had decayed teeth. As one examining dentist said: "The implications for these families are that teeth become decayed, remain untreated, and finally are extracted." In another survey, of National Youth Administration participants in 1941, it was found that each member of the group of sixty thousand had an average of four or five teeth in some stage of decay.

As of June 30, 1943, there were dental programs in 356 counties in 25 states, with a membership of 39,373 families or 201,780 persons. One such program, it was reported in the FSA hearings, was in Colorado where an agreement with the state dental society provided for the dentist to be paid on an hourly basis for usually two scheduled appointments per year per family, at an average annual cost of $8.00. It was also stated that Idaho had one dental unit covering one county, Utah had two plans working in three counties, and Wyoming had three medical plans in three counties that also offered dental care (U.S. Congress, 1943).

Dental Care to Low-Income Utah Farmers. A February 6, 1941, article in the Salt Lake *Tribune* tells of an agreement signed February 5 between the Utah State Dental Association and the Farm

Security Administration, which was to "provide needed dental care for low income farm families by means of cooperative pooling of funds and at a cost within the ability of the families to pay." The plan had previously been approved by the dental association on December 2, 1940. Dr. K. W. Merrill, President of the Utah State Dental Association at the time, was quoted as saying:

> It is expected that the program will begin operating in Cache, Rich, Uintah, Duchesne, Sanpete, and Sevier counties within the next few months. It will be extended to other areas of the state as rapidly as possible. . . . Participation in the plan will be restricted to FSA borrowers. It is expected, however, that similar plans may be extended to the groups of rural families. . . . The dental profession has been constantly seeking some means whereby dental care could be given without depriving individuals of their freedom to choose their own dentists, without injury to the standards of dental care and without the costly intervention of a third party between the dentist and his patient. We feel this progress points the way to a solution.

A succeeding report on February 9 ("Dentists Okey [*sic*] Service Plan," 1941) states that the First District Dental Society, which at that time included Box Elder, Rich, and Cache counties, approved the state plan and also said that it "assures FSA borrowers of complete dental care over a five-year period through a pooling of funds within the ability of each family to pay."

D. Ivo Eames was the district supervisor for the FSA at the time Utah's dental cooperatives began, and later became state supervisor. He remembers that one family's price for dental care was $10 or $12 for the first two years. After that, the price went down some, "as we figured, they [FSA borrowers] would get most of their work done in those first two years." With only so much money in the pool, dentists would not be paid for extra work after a certain point, so the emphasis came to be on prevention, Eames said. "There was always a lot of work to do, so it never worked out that the dentists would get money for services not provided."

Most of the dental services provided were emergency ones, said former Dental Society President Merrill, now retired and living in Preston, Idaho. "I thought it was very successful," he recalls. "We certainly took care of the people who needed help and didn't have the money to pay. The doctors were very cooperative and their attitude was wonderful. The people got the same calibre of dental care as if they had paid for it themselves, and we had no problems with people coming in repeatedly for minor complaints.

"Eventually," said Merrill, "all eight dental districts in the state cooperated under the plan, but as economic conditions improved, people no longer needed help. It died a natural death."[9]

Co-ops Flourished

For a while both the dental and medical plans flourished across the United States, from eight counties in 1936 to a high of 1,131 counties in 1942. If one allows for multi-county units, there were 1,062 different group plans with a combined membership of 116,631 families or 615,985 persons in 42 states and Puerto Rico (Ziegler *et al.*, 1947).

Some doctors were eager to see the FSA medical plans enter their counties; others, like Dr. Schiess's peers, had apprehensions about such plans being the wedge in the door for socialized medicine. Generally, it seemed that the urban doctors who did not have as much experience with the special problems of rural medicine were against the FSA medical plans and believed they would pave the way to socialized medicine, while the country doctors, who knew the situation and were treating patients without payment, were in favor. In the words of a medical society chairman: "Where the program is in operation, they like it, and where they know nothing about it, they are raising hell!" (Hellman, 1940).

Proponents emphasized that since medical care was on a prepayment plan and doctors would get only a certain maximum, no matter how much service they provided, there was a push on preventive medicine. Some physicians would ask all their FSA patients to be home on a certain Saturday and then make their rounds, leaving suggestions and prescriptions. Others sent out notices when innoculation time was due. Many stressed the importance of diet, encouraging farmers to grow vegetable gardens. By 1938, the production of food for the home had tripled.

According to Hellman (1940), before the FSA medical plan was established, it was estimated that the average rural doctor might collect about 50 percent of his bills, with the percentage

[9]Telephone interview, January 8, 1975.

usually between a high of 40 to a low of 20. One Kansas doctor had kept records concerning his payments (Mott and Roemer, 1948) and found that

> ... three years from January 1936 to January 1939, he had collected from 42 families an average of 11 percent of the amount of bills submitted. By individual households, payments varied from zero to a high of 56 percent. The same 42 families later joined up with an FSA medical plan, and the doctor's books show that during the first six months between May and December 1939, he collected 61 percent.

In 1941, this same 61 percent was the national average payment of all doctors' bills, report Mott and Roemer, as was 81 percent for all dentists' bills and 74 percent for all hospitals' bills.

Complaints, Too. Not everyone was happy with FSA medical cooperatives. One borrower, during a visit to a dentist, said that he wanted gold fillings. He was told that gold was not "a part of the bargain" and that amalgam was good enough. "Well," he huffed, "if I can't get a gold tooth, I don't want any. I knew there was a catch in it somewhere" (Goding, 1942).

But there were many legitimate complaints, too. Far too few members actually joined; the turnover was high, with those needing excessive medical care electing to stay in the program. One man said that he wouldn't pay the $16 fee "because on the average, we don't use more than sixteen dollars' doctoring a year, and we don't think we can save by joining" (Goding, 1942). Thus those who needed medical care joined the cooperatives, flooding the doctors with work, and those who didn't require medical attention – but whose fees were crucial to the success of the plan – opted not to join. To make matters worse, because the plans were confined to persons with low income, the amount of money taken in was small, and medical benefits had to be limited. Many of the programs were weak in certain essential aspects of good medical care, such as treatment of the chronically ill, elective surgery, consultations, periodic health examinations, or referrals to specialists either near by or in a distant city or town.

At times there were problems with the fee-for-service payment plan. The more services provided, the lower the percentage of payment for each service, and there was sometimes a tendency by the doctor to reduce the volume of patients. Sharp variations in payment month to month put a stress on the relationship with professional groups. It was difficult, if not impossible, to achieve soundness and stability when memberships, and thus payments, were small.

In addition, there was the attendant problem of lack of technology. Any medical program that limits itself in area also limits itself in technological innovations. And in the case of rural health programs of the 1930s and '40s, physicians were unable to take advantage of urban medical facilities. At other times, there was too little local membership participation in leadership and in the formation of plans, as well as a general lack of supervision. Drugs, too, proved to be a problem to the program and its recipients. Unless the local druggist accepted a pro rata payment or gave a fixed discount, as much as 35 percent of the fund could easily be spent on drugs, where 7 to 12 percent is nearer the normal rate.

Abuse of the program was also a concern, but general consensus seemed to be that while abuse of was almost inevitable, it was not rampant. Often families called on the doctor during the first week to see if the plan really worked. When they found that it did, the orientation phase was over. Yet the reverse was sometimes true: Families were so accustomed to going without a doctor's care that they seldom bothered to call him. During the first seven months of the program, it was found that in one recently organized group 57 percent used their medical plan two times or less (Hellman, 1940).

In some cases, it was the physician who was the charlatan, perhaps by getting families to agree to pay the difference between the original bill and the reduced FSA bill. Another type of chiseling was exemplified by the rural physician's story reported by Lubell and Everett (1938):

> ...[A] farmer came up to me not long ago and said, "Doc, I've got a lot of relatives coming to visit me and I haven't got enough to eat myself. Couldn't you come out to my place — call it a broken arm or anything — and get a few dollars to help me out?" I did it... because I knew he needed it.

Less compassionate cheating included making extra calls to make up for pro-rated bills, faking calls, treating visiting relatives under the names of family members, submitting bills for families not on the program, and charging higher fees for members of FSA families than for others at the same economic level.

The Farm Security Administration Program Declines

During World War II and immediately thereafter, the FSA program declined, primarily because the number of eligible borrowers involved decreased from 60 percent in 1942 to 30 percent in 1946. Prosperity in agriculture began to return, giving farmers a sense of security and economic independence and decreasing their desire – and, many times, their need – to enter the program. A large percentage of the rural doctors and dentists had joined the Armed Forces, increasing the shortage of rural medical personnel (Ziegler *et al.*, 1947). Those who remained earned higher incomes than ever before and were not eager to sign an agreement committing themselves to serve any one group. Doctors were reluctant to see farmers who had paid back their government loans on the program, stating that they were now able to afford their own medical services. The war also depleted the FSA field staff, leaving meager numbers of employees and inexperienced supervisors.

All of these problems, plus the inherent weakness of any program that must rely on voluntary participation, forced the decline of the Farm Security Administration. The fact that fewer farmers were participating in the medical cooperatives, as well as fewer doctors and administrators, brought about its ultimate demise. By 1946, only 951 counties and 36 states and Puerto Rico had active medical cooperatives, including five plans in five Idaho counties, four plans in 22 counties in Montana, eight plans in thirteen counties in Utah, and one each for three Wyoming counties. By this time, all of the medical cooperatives had died out in Colorado.

In August 1946, Congress abolished the Farm Security Administration and established the Farmers Home Administration, giving it the responsibility of administering – but not the authority to organize, manage, or conduct – rural medical programs. Without this authority, it was powerless to keep the moribund medical programs alive (Ziegler *et al.*, 1947).

Yet for more than a decade, the Farm Security Administration's medical cooperatives had helped thousands of people who would have been unable to pay for necessary medical and dental care. These were the nation's rural poor, on the lowest rung of the income ladder, and perhaps the least healthy in all the nation. For them, the FSA plans provided the security that comes from the realization that a bad cold probably won't mean pneumonia and a medical emergency doesn't necessarily mean death.

Selected References

"Dentists Okey Service Plan." Salt Lake *Tribune*, February 9, 1941.

Goding, Harriet Kirk. "Better Health for Farm Families." *Public Health Nursing* (November 1942), vol. 34.

Hellman, Richard. "The Farmers Try Group Medicine." *Harpers* (December 1940), vol. 182.

Lubell, Samuel; and Everett, Walter. "Rehearsal for State Medicine." *Saturday Evening Post* (December 17, 1938).

Mott, F. D.; and Roemer, M. I. *Rural Health and Medical Care*. New York: McGraw-Hill Book Company. 1948.

Rasmusson, A. Vernon. "The Government Work Relief Project in Utah, 1932–1940." Salt Lake City: University of Utah. 1942. Master's thesis.

Salt Lake *Tribune*, February 6, 1941; January 10, 1943.

Stout, Wayne, *History of Utah.* Volume 3. Salt Lake City: Private printing. 1971.

Williams, R. C., M.D. "Development of Medical Care Plans for Low Income Farm Families." *American Journal of Public Health and the Nation's Health* (July 1940), vol. 30, no. 7.

U.S. Congress, House, Committee on Agriculture, *Hearings, Farm Security Administration*, 78th Cong., 1943.

Ziegler, Mark; *et al.* "Rural Prepayment Medical Care Plans and Public Health Agencies." *American Journal of Public Health* (December 1947), vol. 37.

5

Private Medical Cooperatives Come to the Country

Group health plans, which supply basic medical and hospital needs to members, have been in existence in the United States for some time, the oldest probably being the Northern Pacific Railroad Beneficial Association founded in 1822. During the Depression of the 1930s, these plans, like the Farm Security Administration plans, flourished. Poverty, a bitter experience that many faced, induced people to look for ways in which to protect their families' health, even though money was scarce. Hospitals were also in financial trouble, and administrators sought methods to keep their buildings open by maintaining at least a 50 percent occupancy ratio (average at that time).

In 1929, a successful prepaid hospitalization plan for teachers began at Baylor University Hospital in Dallas, Texas. Other hospitals across the nation eagerly adopted the Baylor idea – the forerunner of Blue Cross. But such plans were only a partial answer to the country's medical care problems, for coverage was restricted to the employed, usually white-collar and middle-income groups, their dependents not being covered. Private medical cooperatives for rural residents were less common; but as the idea became more widely accepted and the need more greatly felt, rural people also began uniting for better medical care.

The Elk City Experience

The first rural medical cooperative, located in the dusty plains of western Oklahoma, was not too far from the Intermountain Region. Dr. Michael Shadid, a Syrian physician who had settled in the small town of Elk City, Oklahoma, was a socialist who felt that a group practice and payment plan would bring better health care to the residents of his adopted home. Elk City already had cooperative gins, oil stations, and grocery stores, and the idea of cooperative medicine was enthusiastically received by all the townspeople.

But when Shadid began his plan, group practice was illegal in Oklahoma, as it was in most states. Harassed by the local and state medical societies, Shadid filed a suit which was subsequently ruled in his favor by the state supreme court. The publicity doubtless spurred the development of rural and private medical cooperatives in other states, including those in the Intermountain Area.

The Intermountain West Adopts the Oklahoma Idea

By 1949, there were eight of the Oklahoma-type cooperatives on record in the Intermountain Area (Johnston, 1950): two each in Colorado and Utah and four in Idaho (which had lost three but was in the process of organizing another). Colorado had one prepayment plan (the other was not), and Utah had one prepayment cooperative and one that had been disbanded.

It often took a local emergency to get a medical cooperative started. Or it may be that the people were both aware of and frightened by the fact that the nearest hospital was fifty miles away or that nearer ones were so crowded that beds were in the hallways. Or it may be that residents had trouble paying for their medical bills and liked the idea of prepayment, or had seen successful cooperatives and decided that they could take care of their own needs if only they could form a cooperative association. Whatever the reasons, cooperatives seemed to be the answer for poor people, especially the rural poor.

Rural Utah Recognizes the Need. In 1938, local community leaders of San Juan County, a sprawling area in the southwest corner of Utah, realized that they must do something about health care for their constituents. At that time, the county had no doctors and only one registered nurse to look after the health of the 3,400 people within its borders. If residents in, say, Bluff required a physician's care, they had to travel the hundred miles to Moab, in adjoining Grand County, or sixty miles to San Juan County's largest town, Monticello. Or they could go to Cortez, Colorado, which was ten miles farther. "Lots of babies were born at home, and many broken arms and legs were not set properly," remembers A. J. Redd,[1] a retired banker and merchant living in Monticello. "Many people died for lack of medical attention before we could even get to them."

Monticello's mayor expressed his concern in an article ("A Successful Medical Cooperative Association," 1939):

> I feel that 75 percent of the people of the county and town have not had sufficient medical attention.... The health of our younger generation has been impaired because of the lack of doctors to give periodical examinations.... In the case of a serious accident, it has been necessary to move the patient sixty miles to a doctor, or else wait for the doctor to make the same trip, and this has been the cause of loss of lives. We have had no doctor to take care of maternity cases. This has been done by midwives without license or professional training.

The late David Evans at that time was head of the county Farm Security Administration program and knew of the needs of the people in his jurisdiction. He and others – prominent civic officials, church leaders, and public health agents – devised a cooperative plan out of necessity, according to A. J. Redd. After discussing the idea with Moab's Dr. I. W. Allen and hospital officials in Moab, they determined that people could receive good medical attention if they prepaid a fee of $25 a family into a cooperative association. Of this amount, $15 went to the doctor and $10 to the hospital in Moab. This allowed any family member of the plan to get medical service and hospitalization at $1.00 a day, plus the cost of medication. The money, according to Redd, paid for doctors' services, childbirth, surgery, and most other medical problems. Private enrollment was encouraged, and most found that they could afford low fees; but for FSA borrowers who could not

[1]Telephone interview, January 8, 1975.

afford these fees, their loans were increased to cover the extra amount so that they could join the cooperative.

"It was one of the finest things that ever happened in this county," said Ms. Arvilla Warren,[2] who lived in Monticello and now works in San Juan County's recorder's office. "I was a widow at the time the program started and had two little boys. Then I was newly married, didn't have any insurance, and was really in a panic. When they came to me about joining, I went right out and found my husband and asked him if we could write a check for it. I had a baby on that program, and the care was very personal – Dr. Allen went with me to the hospital and was with me the whole time. I had some complications and was in the hospital fourteen days. When I got the bill, the whole thing came to only twenty-one dollars. And I got the best special care you ever saw."

A. J. Redd was one of the community leaders who helped establish the plan. His family of seven was enrolled. During his telephone interview, he recalled, "Two of our children had polio and spent quite a bit of time in a special wing at St. Mark's Hospital in Salt Lake City. We had to pay for that, as it was outside the county. But previously, they had spent several weeks at the hospital in Moab at a dollar a day. Also, Mrs. Redd had a major operation or two while we were in the program.

"I remember a schoolteacher in Monticello whose wife had two babies in one year on the program. Also, she was stricken with polio, and their children had several tonsilectomies and quite a few minor things taken care of – and this was all in one year."

Abuse Brings on Demise. After the program had been in existence for some time, members started abusing the program, according to Ms. Warren. "Two or three people in each family were getting their appendixes out, and everybody was having their tonsils out whether they needed to or not. The [amount of] care got so great that another doctor, Dr. Austin, came in and lived in Blanding. After he left, Dr. Wesley Bayles moved in to help."

Adds Mr. Redd, "It got to working so well [that] we had to raise the price to fifty dollars a year, and then to seventy-five dollars. As the services of more doctors became available, the program began to seem superfluous. Also, people shied away from the

[2]Telephone interview, January 8, 1975.

seventy-five dollars; and after about five years, the program died out."

Most cooperatives faced at least a few problems, the accumulation of which caused their demise. Some had trouble with the initial financing, and it was difficult to raise money in counties where cooperatives were most needed because while the people were desperate for medical care, they were also desperately poor. Sometimes it turned out that the costs were greater than expected, and it was found that the fee had been set far too low. Since skepticism about a new idea kept many families from joining until they saw substantial evidence that a cooperative could succeed, gaining community support, and hence membership, was immensely difficult.

At other times, community leaders failed to find out what the people really wanted and needed, or there was indifference on the part of the local residents, a lack of understanding about cooperatives, and even rumors of communism. Organizational problems surfaced everywhere. Shortages not only of materials but also of doctors and nurses caused delays or defaults, as did meeting the cost of operation and the opposition from organized medicine. And there was always the problem of keeping the dues low enough to attract members and yet high enough to provide good medical care.

The Telluride Health Association and Dr. Parker

One of the earliest cooperatives in the Intermountain Area – in Telluride, Colorado – didn't have the last problem described above. It was fortunate enough to get excellent care for the astonishingly low fee of $2.00 a month. For this price, families living near the western Colorado mining town could join the Telluride Health Association. All of their medical needs, except obstetrics and general surgery, were provided – and all by one physician and one nurse, Dr. and Mrs. Joseph Parker.

"I went to Telluride in 1932 at the height of the Depression," said Dr. Parker,[3] who now lives in Grand Junction, Colorado. "I had just finished my internship in Tacoma, Washington, and a few bucks were hard to come by. Nobody had any money. And if

[3]Personal interview, April 9, 1975.

[the patients] had a choice of buying a sack of potatoes or paying the doctor bill, you know what [the choice] is, and you really can't blame them for that."

Since money was so scarce Dr. Parker decided to work for the prepaid plan in Telluride, which was established before the Parkers moved there. Dr. Parker received $2.00 per month for each family, which usually came to about $185 per month. He received $25 a month for serving as City Health Officer and another $25 for being County Health Officer, which guaranteed him at least $235 each month. "But I had medical school classmates who were doctors at the CCC camps getting $166 a month – and they thought I had it made as I was getting $235."

But if Dr. Parker "had it made" so far as money was concerned, he seemed indeed to earn his keep. "There was no limit to the amount of times [patients in the program] could call me; and, boy, did they take advantage of me. There was a little work going on at the mine all the time, so I thought that I had to have evening office hours. I had office hours in the morning, office hours in the afternoon, and office hours in the evening until nine p.m. every day. And, my gosh, you ought to have heard those people cry if I took a Saturday night off to have a dinner party or something. And night calls – there was no end to night calls . . . but they were entitled to it.

"I've made house calls and driven as far as ninety miles for deliveries. And at that time, I was charging thirty-five dollars for a delivery. Well, I think for those prairie calls, I charged them about fifteen dollars extra – but I didn't want to charge them too much extra because I didn't want to lose them," he hastened to add. Then he said wryly, "You know, if you charge them thirty-five dollars and you don't get it, you have lost only thirty-five dollars. But if you charge them seventy-five dollars, then you have lost seventy-five dollars."

Transportation in Telluride. The roads that Dr. Parker traveled in making his house calls were "not the best," he said. They wound "up and down the canyons and went around every point and up every draw. Since then, [there are] some nice oiled roads [which] take you right onto the main highway and south to Durango."

Although Dr. Parker always drove a Ford (except in 1936, when he bought a Lincoln Zephyr, which he termed "a lemon"), the train was used by many for transportation. While discussing the railroad between Telluride and Ridgway, Colorado, Dr. Parker's wife[4] described the train as having "a car motor and wheels," and told of the steep hill called Keystone Hill, "It is very steep... and [the train] goes so slow up the hill, you could get off and walk that fast or faster. Once this woman asked the conductor if he couldn't hurry as she was going to have a baby. He said 'Lady, if you're in that condition, you shouldn't have got on the train.' And she said, 'I wasn't in that condition when I first got on this train.' "

The Parkers lived in Telluride for fifteen years, during which time he was the only doctor in town. He also worked this entire time on the prepaid program. "I took care of an area bigger than two or three of the New England states, bigger than Rhode Island and Delaware put together. But, you know, the population was scattered. I think [the number of] people I took care of altogether was about two thousand."

Dr. Parker's Practice. When the Parkers first went to Telluride there were no more than seven hundred or eight hundred people living there. "We had our office in our house for three years. The dining room was the receptionist's room. And I had a little bedroom off that room that was the consultation room or the examining room.... We had no place to do any operations, and we worked for about four years without an X ray. [We] set bones and, by gosh, I was pretty good at it. We'd get a box of plaster... and stretch [the patient] out on the table. She [his wife] would put the leg to sleep... and I'd get the scrub bucket to soak my plaster in and set up the leg and wrap it up."

Ms. Parker, a registered nurse, was her husband's anesthetist for most of his operations. When she was in nurse's training, she was taught the drip-type method of administering ether. Later on, she was told that this method was the safest to use in the high altitudes of the Rocky Mountains. However, as she was relating some of her experiences to a physician in Grand Junction, Colorado, she was chastised as having "no business giving anesthetics" because she had not been trained in anesthesiology. Her reply to that was, "Well, every one of them woke up!"

Spinals were also used. On one occasion, a man with a "hot appendix" that was ready to rupture was given a spinal by Ms. Parker. She asked him to "speak up" when he felt numb enough

---

[4]Personal interview, April 9, 1975.

for the doctor to operate. Added Dr. Parker, "This old guy yelled, 'Jesus Christ, Doctor, you can't operate on me now! I'm not asleep yet!' I explained the spinal to him, but it didn't do any good."

The Parkers often dealt with abortions, both spontaneous and self-induced. "You never knew which one it was, but if they were hemorrhaging, you had to do something about it," said Dr. Parker. "And we'd go down and put them to sleep and scrape them out. Then after we got the hospital, we really went first class – we brought them up and put them on the operating table."

A material often used to induce an abortion was the "slippery elm," a wood that when moistened and inserted into the cervix expands and causes the body to abort the fetus. "I couldn't say who did and who didn't [use the device], but the druggist told me he sold an awful lot of slippery elms. It wasn't his business to ask them what they wanted it for."

During their first winter in Telluride, when the snow was "deeper than hell," a man came to Dr. Parker badly scalded. When asked how it happened, he replied that his chicken boiler had blown up. Said Dr. Parker, "Well, I've had a little experience with chickens, but I have never seen a hot-water-heated chicken boiler, and anyone who was raising chickens in February was nuts. But I didn't question him at all and later found out that he had let his still get boiling a little too heavy, and it boiled the mash up into the coils, and that had plugged the coils. He had no relief valve on the boiler, and the dang thing exploded – and that is how he was scalded."

His first amputation was also the result of an alcohol-related incident. "Someone had just happened to notice a light ten or twelve feet from the main pathway through the snow. A fellow had passed out drunk there, and his hand was frozen tight to the flashlight. But it was still lighted, and that was what called someone's attention. They brought him in, and we actually had to thaw his hands out to get them away from the flashlight. I don't remember how many fingers he did lose."

The Parkers also recounted the story about the time Ms. Parker was delivering a baby but had no string with which to tie the cord. She took a shoe string from one of the doctor's shoes and got the job done. Another time, she herself was in labor with their second son when a small boy with appendicitis was brought to the doctor. She had to get out of bed to help with the anesthetic. "She'd give some to the kid, then she'd take some herself," added the doctor.

"I've wondered how in the heck we practiced medicine in those days without the drugs we have today — no sulfa, no antibiotics, no tranquilizers, no antihistamines. And they are all good drugs if properly used." And while medicines have improved, Dr. Parker feels that medical care has not. "You can't get a doctor that will go into these small areas and work. No, the mining company at Telluride [today] has to pay a doctor quite a subsidy just to keep him there, and they also furnish [the doctor] with a first-class clinic. Hell, I didn't have anything that I didn't buy myself, including the operating table.... I was the only one up there. And I never turned down a call. Sometimes I'd be up all night long with a mine blast or something. And then I'd have to work the next day because I had things to do. And then the next night, I had to go again lots of times. No one else [was there to] relieve you, you just had to go."

There were times when patients called him from other communities, wanting to know if they could come to the office. He would tell them that the office closed at 9:00 p.m.; but if they weren't able to get there before the closing hour, he made "a call to their house and wouldn't return until midnight. Most of the nights when the phone would ring, I'd pick up the receiver and hear the compressor, and they didn't even have to say a word because [I knew] they were calling from the mine and, according to the miners and other people, I'm the last doctor that ever went into the mine. But whenever anyone was fiercely hurt, I'd go into the mine and give him some morphine, splint his leg or whatever to make his move more comfortable. We had to ride the aerial trams, basically the same as ski lifts today. But these were buckets that held about a thousand pounds of ore. You just got in the bucket and rode up."

Vacations were rare for the rural doctor at that time. "From 1936 to 1946 we were never out of Telluride as much as twenty-four hours. That was [during the] ten years I couldn't get relief. And then the war came on, and a vacation was strictly out of the question."

Today, an oft-heard objection about a doctor's going into rural practice is lack of time away from the office and from care of his patients. But the wives have a complaint, too — the isolation from cultural events and from friends. However, Ms. Parker felt none of this. "We were so busy that we didn't have time to be lonely. We had to make our own amusements... and we had a supper club and we played bridge." Because she had been raised in a strictly religious Luthern household, "there wasn't a deck of cards in our house because that was the devil's bible. I didn't know one suit from the other, and this little lady [in Telluride] tried to teach me."

There were other types of entertainment to be found. Telluride, before it became the ski area it is today, and before there were ski lifts, was a ski enthusiast's ideal place, and the Parkers often went skiing there with friends. On one Sunday outing, however, Ms. Parker broker her leg. Said Dr. Parker, recalling the incident, "We always used to take a tubfull of chili and a kettleful of hot dogs and a couple of jugs of whiskey; and it was just about time for lunch.... I said, 'Look, we don't want to break up the party right at dinner time. Why don't we make you comfortable in the back seat of this car and eat lunch with the bunch, and then we'll go in and take care of your leg.' So we did that, and I came back and she was still comfortable but chilling a bit."

"And not very hungry, I'll have you know," added Ms. Parker.

"So I said," continued her husband, "I'm going up the hill just once more and come down, and then we'll set your leg and take care of it." But on his way down the slope, Dr. Parker had an accident – he ran into a tree stump and gashed his leg.

"And then," said Ms. Parker, "we broke up the party."

Selected References

Follman, J. F., Jr. *Medical Care and Health Insurance*. Homewood, Illinois: Richard D. Irwin, Inc. 1963.

Hellman, Richard. "The Farmers Try Group Medicine." *Harpers* (December 1940), vol. 182.

Johnston, Helen L. *Rural Health Cooperatives*. Washington, D.C.: U.S. Department of Agriculture. 1950.

————. "Rural Health Cooperatives." *Public Health Reports* (October 27, 1950), vol. 65, no. 43.

"A Successful Medical Cooperative Association." *Utah Farmer* (January 10, 1939).

6

Organized Medicine Focuses on the Rural Scene

As the Great Depression faded away and World War II came to an end, rural residents in the Intermountain Region began hoping that they could forget the hard times and return to a peaceful, prosperous life. But these two momentous events in the nation's history had caused them to experience things, both good and bad, that they would never forget. One of the good experiences was the public health programs that had given them a taste of what proper, consistent medical care could do for them. Another was the exposure to medical care that was a fringe benefit of being a G.I. These two programs left many with the knowledge that something was wrong with the minimal health care so common in rural areas and that perhaps a physician should not be a luxury only for the cities' well-to-do.

People now had time to think about less tangible matters than surviving a depression or fighting a war. They had time to ponder their lack of good health care, and it became increasingly apparent that there were wide discrepancies in urban and rural health care and, consequently, in health itself. Urban residents had access to more and better health facilities, advanced techniques of specialists, and more health care personnel. Without medical personnel and facilities, rural residents might as well have been living in the days of the purgers and bleeders.

Recognition of Rural Health Problems

The existence of these problems was at last recognized by national health officials and organizations in 1945. The Associated Women of the Farm Bureau Federation had for some time been concerned with the health of their members and other rural people. They issued a formal invitation to the American Medical Association to join with them in a study of the rural health problem and its solution. The AMA responded by establishing a national committee (now council) on rural health.

"The purpose of that committee was to get more doctors and more medical care into the rural areas," says Dr. Fred A. Humphrey,[1] a general practitioner in Fort Collins, Colorado, and one of the original members. "The trustees of the AMA felt that they should do something about it. Our first conference was held in Chicago [March 30, 1949], and each state medical society appointed representatives."

Not all of the states in the Intermountain Area were represented, however, because state medical societies were asked to pay the expenses of their representatives, and some could not afford to do so. Colorado sent three representatives, including Dr. Humphrey, who was on the Colorado State Medical Society Board of Trustees. Utah sent Dr. Kenneth B. Castleton of Salt Lake City; and Dr. E. M. Gans of Harlowton, Montana, represented that state.

The first chairman of the committee, Dr. Franklin Crockett of Lafayette, Indiana, was selected by the members of the AMA. He spoke briefly about the first meeting (Crockett, 1953):

> ... [It] was not a meeting of physicians to solve a health problem. It was a meeting of physicians and laymen to discuss and solve their mutual health problems – tacit recognition that rural health is a job for the citizen and that it requires community cooperation. The conference was national in scope – some 3,500 invitations were extended to all groups thought interested in the problem. Nearly every state was represented.... The ground rules for the conference called for an open forum in which everyone was free to express his opinions. It was believed that through a multitude of ideas a more complete picture would evolve. The conference was exploratory,

[1]Telephone interview, July 23, 1975.

with no preconceived ideas to be supported. Discussion from the floor was deemed important, equal to the prepared addresses.

After the initial conference, an advisory committee was selected from some of the large farm organizations, such as the Farm Bureau, the Grange, the Cooperative Milk Producers Federation, the Farmers Union, and the Farm Foundation of Chicago, for in Dr. Humphrey's opinion, "If you want to do anything with rural people, you'd better have representatives on the committee."

As chairman of the committee, Dr. Crockett had selected physicians to represent each region of the United States. The states of Colorado, Utah, Wyoming, Idaho, Montana, Arizona, and New Mexico were represented by Colorado's Dr. Humphrey. He served on the committee for fifteen years, three of which were as its chairman (after Dr. Crockett stepped down). During the time Humphrey was active on the national council, he also served as chairman of the Colorado State Rural Health Committee and as president of the Colorado State Medical Society.

"It's difficult to say what the National Council on Rural Health accomplished," said Dr. Humphrey during the interview, "but it was and is a good program. Kansas had a plan to get physicians into the rural areas, and we copied that somewhat. We tried to encourage medical schools to put family practitioners on their teaching staffs and to [establish] courses for family practitioners. All this was accomplished since the committee started. Don't say that we alone accomplished it. But we helped bring improvements about, and we brought the subject of rural health to the attention of the general public, the newspapers, physicians, and medical school."

This public exposure helped in the creation of state rural health committees throughout the country and in bringing about many regional health conferences. The first regional conference in the Intermountain Area was held in Logan, Utah, in 1957, according to Dr. Humphrey, with the second regional conference shortly thereafter in Denver.

In 1957, Reed Farnsworth, M.D., was chairman of Utah's Rural Health Committee. In his report on the conference in Logan, he states (Utah State Medical Association, 1957):

> Unquestionably the most prized achievement of this committee during the past year was our assignment as host

> to the Intermountain District Study Conference of the Rural Health Council of the AMA. This district comprises the states of Montana, Wyoming, Utah, Colorado, and New Mexico, and is represented on the council by Dr. F. A. Humphrey of Fort Collins, Colorado. [Dr. Humphrey has stated that he also represented Idaho and Arizona.]... This conference was held on the campus of [Utah State University]... and, despite rigorous weather conditions, served its purpose very well. The importance of this meeting was evidenced by the attendance of Dr. F. C. Crockett, vice president of the AMA, who is chairman of the Council on Rural Health of the AMA; Aubrey Gates, field director; and Dr. F. A. Humphrey, Regional Council representative of the Intermountain Area. All states were represented with the exception of Montana, and a comprehensive program was presented, including seminars, panel discussion, and group participation meetings, resulting in more intimate analysis of our rural health problems. Registration records revealed that some 62 key people participated in the conference.

As public exposure increased, the heightened awareness that resulted precipitated efforts of various organizations and individuals to find a "cure" for the rural health problem.

Government Involvement

Not long after the 1945 recognition of the rural need for medical care personnel and facilities, the federal government became involved in helping to find the solution. In 1946, Congress enacted the Hospital Survey and Construction Act, better known as the Hill-Burton bill, which emphasized construction of hospitals in rural areas. The intent of the Act was twofold (U.S. Department of Health, Education, and Welfare, 1971): "(1) to assist the states in surveying the needs of hospitals and assisting in comprehensive planning for hospital construction, and (2) to provide assistance in financing needed construction."

Funding for the health facilities grant program was based largely on a formula determined by population, weighted by allotment percentage (representing per capita income) squared, or on the need for modernization and new construction of facilities. The federal matching share could be as much as two-thirds of allowable total costs. Eligibility for funding was open to state and local governments, Hill-Burton state agencies, project sponsors, hospital districts or authorities, and other representatives of the hospital community.

Some people were against the Hill-Burton bill, however. In Utah, for example, Dr. Castelton, president of the Salt Lake Medical Society, was quoted as saying ("National Conference on Rural Health," June 8, 1946):

> We need more hospitals or more beds. We need more hospitals where distances are great and doctors scarce. People in Utah don't want federal money for this; they are not interested in the Hill-Burton bill. The [Mormon] church offered help for supplying different hospitals needed. Several hospitals were built and maintained by the Mormon Church. This plan is endorsed by the Utah State Medical Society and we hope it will fill our hospital needs without calling on federal funds.

But by June 30, 1973, not only had 77 Hill-Burton projects been approved in Utah, there were also 125 approved in Colorado, 92 in Idaho, 99 in Montana, 49 in Nevada, and 66 in Wyoming, many of which were in rural areas. These statistics alone, taken from the U.S. Department of Health, Education, and Welfare, Office of Planning and Analysis's "Facts about the Hill-Burton Program" (no date), attest to the vast need for hospitals in rural, suburban, and urban areas of the Intermountain West.

In 1964, however, the Act was amended to establish a new program for the modernization or replacement of public and nonprofit hospitals and other health facilities. The 1964 Hill-Harris amendments switched the emphasis from farms (which the original Hill-Burton bill had advocated) to the cities, giving consideration to facilities in more densely populated areas where the greatest need was thought to exist. The Hill-Burton Act helped the rural areas at first, but the same thing happened to it as to most of the other 1950s and '60s rural health programs. They lasted for a time and then gradually diminished in importance as either the program itself or the people behind it withdrew from the scene.

Dr. Florence Rena Sabin's Crusade

Individuals also took part in the crusade for improved rural health in the Intermountain Region. Among these, the name of

Florence Rena Sabin stands out. She was the first woman to earn a doctorate in medicine from Johns Hopkins University, the first woman professor on its faculty, and the first woman member of the Rockefeller Institute for Medical Research. In addition, she'd had twelve honorary degrees bestowed upon her. When in 1938 she retired from the Rockefeller Institute at age 67, she sought the mountains of Colorado.

Colorado at that time had done little to aid rural residents in their quest for medical care. As late as 1947, the Denver Health and Charity Department was housed at the end of a long corridor in the county hospital – it wasn't even listed in the telephone directory. According to Kauver *et al.* (1950): "That Denver does not have a good local health department is too obvious to warrant comment. It might truthfully be said that Denver does not have a health department at all in the commonly accepted sense of the term."

The Denver Health and Charity Department, by virtue of the city's being the largest in Colorado and one of the larger in the United States, would seemingly have had a sound health program. Instead, it had no professional leadership, no civil service or merit system for health care personnel, no full-time medical personnel (qualified or unqualified), and not even an adding machine for the vital statistics section of the department. The manager of the overall department was not only responsible for the duties implied by his title, he was also director of the Denver General Hospital and the "county poor farm." He served as the coroner, was responsible for garbage collection, and occasionally served subpoenas. With Colorado's largest city in such utter confusion so far as its health care was concerned, one could hardly expect the remainder of the state to be in better circumstances to take care of its sick. It wasn't.

In 1944, Governor John Vivian drew up a list of names of people who could qualify as appointees to a postwar planning committee which was to help remedy the situation. When he showed the list to Frances Wayne, a reporter for the local newspaper (the Denver *Post*), she wasted few words upon seeing that no women's names were included. The governor asked for her suggestions and she told him of Dr. Sabin. Thus, as a token to women's interests, the subcommittee on health was headed by the 73-year-old retired Dr. Sabin.

It is possible that Governor Vivian thought that Dr. Sabin's appointment would upset few political applecarts because of the quiet life she had been leading since coming to Colorado. But Dr. Sabin turned out to be an extraordinarily capable woman who found many things wrong with the state's medical services and set out to change them. Her first act was to obtain a grant from the Commonwealth Fund of New York City. Dr. Carl Buck of the American Public Health Association was sent to Colorado to make a study of the state's health laws and disease-fighting facilities.

The report, submitted to the subcommittee on health in January 1946, showed that the prevailing theory of "Colorado as a health resort" was in actuality a myth. In fact, 34 states and the District of Columbia had better records than Colorado in deaths due to preventable or controllable disease. Only two states had worse rates for scarlet fever; only five were worse than Colorado in diphtheria; and 41 states had better records for diarrhea enteritis and pneumonia fatalities. Infant mortality was higher than all except seven states. In the five years prior to the study, 14,662 Coloradoans had died from preventable and controllable diseases. If what was known about preventive medicine at that time had been applied, 8,245 of those dead could possibly have been saved. More than three times as many Coloradoans died of these diseases as Colorado lost during all of World War II (Maisel, 1947).

Dr. Buck's study found that Colorado was giving its Division of Public Health less than ten cents per capita to protect its citizens' health. The division managed to survive on pitifully small sums from the U.S. Public Health Service and the Children's Bureau. State appropriations to health care were only 14 percent of the total, less than half as much as Montana contributed to its program, and less than a third of Utah's percentage (Maisel, 1947).

The Division of Public Health was politically controlled, and the Civil Service Commission had been blocking the appointment of qualified health officials. Six of the chief administrative positions in the state's health agency were vacant. Salaries were 26 percent lower in Colorado than in the surrounding states. In addition, only five of Colorado's 63 counties could boast a local health department; three of the five were without full-time health officers.

Most localities in the state had never undertaken the health-protecting functions that were commonplace in nearly every area of the United States. There was no effective control over the milk supply, and the health division had no authority to regulate milk production or dairy herds. Only two counties and nine towns were operating under the standard milk ordinance of the U.S. Public Health Service. Barely half of the communities in the state had pollution-free water, and only 16 percent had modern sewage systems. In the entire state, nearly half of the localities had no sewer system whatsoever; others had systems incapable of purifying water before it was dumped into streams where it could pollute irrigation water and contaminate truck farming crops (Maisel, 1947).

For generations, tuberculosis victims throughout the United States had been coming to Colorado's renowned sanitaria. But the investigation found that TB was rampant among Colorado's own residents, with a mere 574 beds available to them – less than half the minimum number required. Said Dr. Sabin (1947):

> Two different types of work were then started, both closely correlated with each other: first, the organization of an executive committee for intensive study of the report and for drawing up the bills to be presented to the legislature; and second, the carrying out of Dr. Buck's report and the Health Committee's plans as they developed directly to the people of the state.

Members of the executive committee had many long meetings, inviting representatives of groups that would be affected by the proposed development of health services. But they also invited "experts" who could give advice, thus forestalling opposition.

One victory was the winning of support of members of the dairy industry. Many conferences were held with them. At one point, Dr. Sabin asked why they opposed the program, inviting them to have a representative on the health committee. They eventually appointed a man who, according to Dr. Sabin (1947),

> ...gave much help and arranged conferences with members of the Dairy Association, and with all the experts on the subject of milk in Colorado, both from the federal and state groups. Full agreement was reached on the need for higher standards and improved practices for production and for processing of milk and milk products.

Later on, the governor appointed both a milk processor and a milk producer to the Colorado State Board of Health, enabling the health department and the dairy industry to work together (Sabin, 1947).

Because popular support was vital to the successful passage of state health laws which the committee had begun to formulate, Dr. Sabin made a whirlwind tour of Colorado, telling the populace of the dismal amount of health protection it now suffered, but also giving the people a ray of hope that something could be done about it.

She spoke before PTA groups, men's clubs, medical associations, farmers' meetings, and groups of interested lay people, always paying her own way for the sometimes perilous trips through the snows of the Rockies. According to Maisel (1947):

> Many who come to hear her are at first drawn more by curiosity than by an avid interest in public health. Their first shock comes as she begins to excoriate "unnecessary death." She has the ability to make figures come to life. When she talks of babies made sick by tainted milk, mothers feel she is talking of their own babies. Her intolerance toward contagion is itself contagious.

Data on the local and state health conditions were presented at these meetings. Discussions were held on how public health action could effect changes, but initiation of action was left to the people. The first response was a fund for a sewage disposal plant, started in a town where raw sewage was dumped into the river. In another community, women told of milk too dirty to use. The supervisor of nurses and the town's manager met with the women and the health committee in Colorado Springs, where an impeccably run dairy and a superb pasteurization plant were observed. The visitors were so impressed that they asked two dairies to ship pasteurized milk to their town. It wasn't long before a local dairy established its own pasteurization plant.

Seven bills drawn up by the executive committee on health were eventually passed in the state legislature. The state reorganization bill created the Colorado Department of Public Health, with a board of health and an executive division. The mandate to the executive division was that it set up county, city-county, and multi-county health units. Two appropriations bills were also passed – one for the department itself and the county units, and the other for the medical school. An enabling act to allow federal requirements for participation in the Hill-Burton plan was approved, as were two special bills to lessen the incidence of tuberculosis: (1) by increasing per diem allotments to hospitals, and (2) by building thirty additional hospital beds (Sabin, 1947).

Medical Schools Join In

Medical schools across the United States heard the pleas for help from farmers and physicians alike and began looking for ways to aid the hapless rural families. The schools sponsored programs to build hospitals and clinics in small towns, hoping that physicians would be attracted by the new facilities. Some started loan programs for those who wanted to become rural doctors. Others considered traveling clinics to treat patients who otherwise would not take the time from planting and harvesting to make the trip to a doctor.

In the Intermountain Region, only two states, Utah and Colorado, had medical schools. Thus a vast amount of rural areas was unable to receive medical school help. But some rural residents did receive assistance from the University of Utah College of Medicine in Salt Lake City and the University of Colorado Medical Center in Denver.

Dr. Kenneth B. Castleton, dean emeritus of the University of Utah College of Medicine, recalls some of the efforts of that school in assisting with rural health care[2]: "At first, there wasn't very much of anything done to improve rural health, except that we did try to take as many candidates for medical school as possible from the rural areas. We wouldn't take a lesser qualified rural person over a more qualified city person, of course, but we talked with them and if they wanted to go into rural practice, we gave them a little plus. And we talked to their wives and found out where they were from, as that was very important."

He also recalls that the AMA gave a "few scholarships" to those who showed an interest in rural medicine, "but it was never a significant number. It seems to me that one student from Utah got one."

Doctors were sent into Indian areas, according to Dr. Castleton. "We had an ear, nose, and throat man and an orthopedist who went quite regularly to treat the Indians in the southern part of the state."

---

[2]Telephone interview, January 29, 1975.

In the 1950s, the Utah medical school put into effect three plans to help the country practitioners. Because overworked rural doctors had little time to read medical literature and few if any chances to find a replacement so that they could attend refresher courses at the university, the medical school began sending out teams of medical men from the university to teach seminars in Utah and parts of Arizona, with funds provided by state medical associations and the Kellogg Foundation. An account of such medical teams tells of a representative journey ("Medical Missionaries," February 16, 1953):

> On the most recent junket, a typical day's drive took Dr. John F. Waldo (internal medicine), Dr. Ralph C. Richards (surgery), and Dr. Richard Burton (obstetrics) 262 miles from Salt Lake City to Cedar City in Utah's red cliff country. The subject of the meeting was "the management of emergencies." The place was a brace of rooms in the verandaed, yellow brick El Escalante Hotel. "We've conducted these meetings in church basements, hotels and motels, very rarely in hospitals," Dr. Waldo noted.

At this meeting, Dr. Richards outlined advances in diagnosis and management of surgical emergencies. Dr. Burton discussed new and simplified laboratory tests that could easily be carried out in the lab facilities to which most of the doctors had access. Dr. Waldo concentrated on antibiotics and their use in preventing infection.

In another session, the medical team used as headquarters the town of Price in the heart of Utah's bituminous coal mining country. Here they met with twenty of the 24 doctors practicing in the vastnesses of Grand, Carbon, and San Juan counties, Utah's canyonlands area. "We were worried when the doctor from Moab showed up," Dr. Waldo recalled. "He left Grand County without a physician for most of the day" ("Medical Missionaries," 1953).

There were reciprocal benefits, however, for as Dr. Waldo said, "While we are dispensing knowledge, we are learning, too. Members of our 'teams' are gaining a new knowledge of the problems of rural practitioners and are thus able to aim our own college curriculum at the Intermountain Area's needs" ("Medical Missionaries").

The second plan of the University of Utah College of Medicine was to beam postgraduate lectures over a local television station to several hospitals in Utah and southern Idaho. The lectures "were of the Wednesday morning surgical grand rounds and of the Thursday medical grand rounds," says Dr. Castleton. "We didn't really go from room to room . . . [the lectures] were held in a classroom and we presented papers and showed patients and X rays. The doctors would get together in their little hospitals [in the outlying areas] and watch and then call in questions."

In 1954, the medical school tried another technique for getting up-to-date medical information to physicians in remote areas. Kits of audiovisual materials were mailed to them, each kit containing 35mm slides (27 to 52 to a kit), a tabletop viewer, and a printed copy and a recording of the lecture. The recording had been taped by a local Salt Lake City firm. Employees in the university's carpenter shops had made the cases which held the slides and records. These cases were cushioned inside to prevent damage to the fragile materials. The tabletop viewers were standard desk models, and the slides were prints of photos taken by the college medical photographer, for a cost of $225 for the master disc, plus slides for each seminar. Copies could be made for $60 a kit ("Doctors Up to Date," 1954).

The kits were disseminated to rural practitioners through the relay method: Four to six doctors were the first to receive a kit and use it. They then mailed it on to other doctors, enabling 550 physicians to receive a postgraduate course for the price of the postage. A typical kit, prepared by Dr. Andrew Latteier, instructor in obstetrics and gynecology at the college, contained 27 slides that took 36 minutes of viewing time. They dealt with the diseases of women's reproductive organs, the cervix, and the vulva ("Doctors Up to Date").

Officials at the University of Colorado Medical Center became concerned about rural health problems when in 1947 Ward Darley was named dean at this Denver school. According to Dr. C. Wesley Eisele,[3] former associate dean for postgraduate education and currently an emeritus and visiting professor at the University of Colorado Medical Center, "Darley grew up in rural Colorado and was quite concerned with rural health. He had teaching teams go out to meet the doctors once a month in various rural parts of the state and see teaching cases. Two doctors would go together and the local doctors would bring in patients related to the subject of

[3]Telephone interview, February 3, 1975.

the day. It was not a clinic where they treated patients, but was for the benefit of the doctors."

From 1947 until the early 1970s, the university maintained an active general practitioner residency through which doctors rotated among rural hospitals, spending three months at each one. "They went to places like Fort Collins and Boulder," says Dr. Eisele, "the smaller communities away from the university. When it became part of the family practice residency, however, the rotating internship was discontinued."

Sears, Roebuck Seeks Solutions

Corporate interests, too, found themselves working for better rural health. During the mid-1950s the Sears, Roebuck Foundation became interested in the problems of medical manpower distribution and asked the AMA for assistance. The AMA appointed a 17-member medical advisory board to the Foundation, and in 1957 the board devised the Community Medical Assistance Plan, a program whose theory was that if more clinics were built, rural areas would be able to attract doctors. According to Moser (January 1965):

> The purpose of the Foundation program is to aid a community and surrounding trade area with a population of 1,500 to 3,000 in obtaining a doctor. The plan includes these facets: (1) an economic survey of a community, using questions drawn up by the Community Medical Assistance Plan but conducted by a nonbiased unit such as the local chamber of commerce or a service organization; (2) a medical center which the residents of the community build and rent for a moderate fee to a doctor or doctors, with option for the lessee to buy; and (3) business and financial counseling and guidance, but no actual financial assistance.

The Sears, Roebuck Foundation program, because of its self-help concept, stipulated that a town must recognize its health problem, must wish to support a doctor, and must provide suitable facilities. After a town had expressed interest and a survey had been taken, and after it was determined that the community showed sufficient potential to support a physician, a town meeting was called. At the meeting, the program was explained, the survey results discussed and, following a question and answer period, a secret ballot taken by the townspeople to decide whether they would participate in the program.

A medical center resulting from these meetings was not financed by the Foundation; only architectural plans were provided, and the community raised the funds necessary to build the clinic. The Foundation, however, helped in the campaign to raise money and in the organization of a trusteeship or a nonprofit corporation to own and manage the building. The structure, designed with a circular patient flow, had a laboratory, an X ray, a dark room, emergency room, four examination-treatment rooms, two consultation rooms, and a central business and reception area sufficient for two doctors. The state medical society and the placement agency of the AMA assisted the local university in finding a physician.

As the final part of the plan, the Foundation provided the services of a professional management consultant to assist the doctor in the business aspects of his practice. This included arranging for financial assistance, guidance in purchasing medical equipment, and business advice.

During the existence of the program from 1958 to 1970, a total of 625 communities completed the survey, and 253 communities were accepted into the program by the Sears, Roebuck Foundation. According to a follow-up study by Kane *et al.* (1973), few applicants came from the medically underserved West. In all, 32 Intermountain Area towns applied, of which, thirteen were rejected and only fourteen built clinics.

The Carbondale Clinic. One of the fourteen towns that built clinics in the Intermountain Region was Carbondale, Colorado, a mining town with a population of 441 in 1958. In February of that year, the townspeople contacted the Sears, Roebuck Foundation to seek its help. The Foundation survey found that an average of fourteen patients a day was traveling to towns from fourteen to thirty miles away for medical care. These Carbondale residents were spending $16,000 annually on doctors' fees and $14,000 on medicine they bought while in those other towns. In addition, they spent $3,500 for fuel to make the trip and $32,000 for nonmedical purchases while there. This amounted to a $65,000 economic loss each year for Carbondale (Furlong, 1958).

Medical help near the mining town was not always of the first magnitude. Carbondale had recently suffered two mine accidents with high fatality rates. The residents complained of poor service when they reached a physician. A contractor whose index finger was severed was forced to drive fourteen miles to a doctor, and then had to wait four hours in the doctor's office before he was treated. People felt frustrated and wanted a doctor in their own town: "When my son was sick last spring, I called up four doctors in towns around here and none would come to see him," said a Carbondale woman. "I finally had to bundle him up and take him to a doctor in Glenwood Springs" (Furlong, 1958).

Plans for the fund-raising drive were outlined in the basement of the Methodist church, and within four months the needed $18,000 for the clinic was raised.

"We established a board and then went from house to house to get the money," said W. H. Harlan,[4] a Carbondale veterinarian who spearheaded the drive. This board is still in charge of managing the clinic and elected by the people at a special election.

The first doctor at "Carbondale's Tri-County Medical Center" was Harry O. Hendricks, a Cincinnati physician who heard about Carbondale during a Colorado vacation. He stayed until about 1971, when he moved to Nevada. "The clinic was empty for about a year," says Harlan. "We just got on the problem and started writing to medical societies and advertising in medical journals. Someone had heard of a doctor in Redbone, Dr. A. T. Waski, who had a summer home there, so the board wrote to him and he moved in. Then in January we got another doctor – Richard Herrington. Both seem to like it here. Herrington says this is where he wants to raise his family. This is a sporting area – there's fishing, hunting, and skiing at both Aspen and Glenwood, and that might have helped us get our doctors."

Carbondale still owns the clinic and rents it to Waski and Herrington. An addition, finished in 1974, is large enough to accommodate three doctors. "We collected the money the same way the second time," says Harlan, "by going door to door. Only this time, prices had gone up so much that we needed a lot more money. We got the biggest part from the people, and the rent on the clinic takes care of the rest."

Demise of the Plan. While the plan was a success in Carbondale, it was not always so effective, and this caused its demise. The follow-up study done by Kane *et al.* (1973) said:

---

[4]Telephone interview, February 21, 1975.

> The project had been in existence for 13 years when the Foundation reevaluated its priorities in 1970 and was discouraged by the fact that one-third of the built clinics were unoccupied. Faced with increasing construction costs, perennial recruitment and retention of frustrations, and a feeling that the project had not been successful for public relations for the parent company, the Foundation decided to discontinue the project. The AMA decided not to assume responsibility and the project was phased out.

Executive director of the Sears, Roebuck Foundation, Ed Quinn,[5] says that it was getting too difficult to attract physicians to justify continuation of the project. "In some ways the program was attracting and holding more doctors than the few comparable programs, but from our point of view it was just getting too difficult. And we might be leading a lot of these towns into a large financial investment that might not have a good return on it."

At the time of Kane's study, of the 253 communities accepted, clinics were built at 165 (65 percent); 163 were successful in obtaining one or more physicians. At the time of follow-up, 132 (81 percent) had at least one physician working in the clinic. In addition, ten other clinics were being used for medical purposes; three were staffed by nurse practitioners or physicians' assistants. In summary, 132 of 253 (52 percent) still had physicians and 142 were still providing medical services to rural residents.

Country Schools Help Rural Health

Another group that helped to reach some of the rural residents were the public schools, a convenient place to reach country youths. Rural and sparsely populated Wyoming used two plans in particular. Michaelson (1971) tells us in the following paragraphs about a program that started in 1954 in Casper, with the hope of diminishing the incidence of rheumatic fever. Brought on by the same germ that causes "strep throat," it usually strikes those between the ages of five and fifteen and is the most common cause of heart disease in children. About three out of every hundred strep throat infections leads to rheumatic fever, which kills fourteen thousand every year. Yet this can be prevented if the streptococcus infections are detected early.

---

[5]Telephone interview, January 29, 1975.

Brenden Phibbs, an internist and former Chicagoan was one of the main forces behind the plan that soon affected 90 percent of Wyoming's schools. He felt it was impossible to detect strep throat by physical examination only and therefore helped instigate a program of mass throat swabbing across the state.

His plan was made possible by a small army of volunteers, usually mothers who had children in school. They came early each morning to their assigned schoolbuilding, laid out the equipment of swabs, flashlight, tongue depressors and record sheets, and waited for the children to arrive.

It became a matter of routine for the teacher to ask the first thing in the morning if any of the children had colds or sore throats. Those who nodded "yes" were sent off to be examined, as was one row per classroom per day, so that all children would get at least a weekly inspection. Kindergarten children, the most susceptible age group, made the trip twice each week.

The children stood in line, some giggling, some squirming, a few practicing their "ahs" ahead of time. But most waited solemnly for their turn. Then they opened their mouths wide, and the trained volunteers inspected the throats. Suspicious throats were deftly swabbed – a harmless but not very gentle looking procedure, as gagging must be produced to get a good moist sample.

A doctor (Michaelson, 1971) told of an incident concerning Dr. Phibbs, which makes him look like the villain of the swabbing crew. A team of physicians were making an at-random check at a school just outside Casper. Dr. Phibbs and two local doctors were sharing duties; it didn't take Phibbs long to acquire a reputation and soon there was not one customer before him. "But when the swabs were cultured," said the storyteller, "he had ninety percent of the positive pickups."

With all throats inspected, the swabs were numbered and listed on a corresponding sheet and delivered to a lab either in Casper or in Cheyenne. There, teams of four would process sometimes more than fifteen hundred swabs each day. Results were given to the school early the next morning and any children found infected with strep were sent home with a note and not allowed to return until treatment had begun.

Results proved gratifying. For example, an Asian flu epidemic hit Wyoming in 1957–58 causing a great outbreak of strep infections. Twenty-five cases of rheumatic fever developed in the general population, but only four cases occurred in the fourteen thousand schoolchildren that were in the program at that time. Normally, 80 percent of this group would be expected to get rheumatic fever.

The Role of the Public Health Nurse

Public health nurses who travel from school to school across the vast Wyoming terrain can also be an influence on the health of rural school children. These nurses see youngsters who, because of the great distances involved and winter blizzards, seldom see a doctor unless there is an extreme emergency.

Jan Miner was a public health nurse in Albany County during the early 1960s (Miner, 1965). Although Albany County is the home of the state's third largest city (Laramie), it is largely rural with scattered ranches. Miner's job was to visit all of the schools in the county that did not employ a full-time health nurse of their own. She would check vision and hearing, talk over problems with teachers and parents, and help set up health teaching projects tailored to the specific problems in each school. The equipment Miner needed was in her car – health teaching aids, audiometer, Snellen charts, plus extra gasoline, water, and a map of Albany County.

Most of the schools were located on or near individual ranches, and Miner drove miles to reach them. To reach ten schools in the Laramie peak area for instance, she traveled 305 miles, much of it on dirt and gravel roads, with sagebrush and cattle often her only company. One trip took her down a rocky canyon, and she had to get out of her car three times to open wire fences. The two students she saw had a new teacher; their last teacher had been frozen to death in a blizzard. In fact, it was the severe weather that mandated all of Miner's school visits be made during late September or early October.

All the ranch schools were grade schools. Once a youngster reached high school age, the school district either provided transportation to school, paid room and board for the student near a high school, or paid an allowance for the family to move. In most cases it was one of the latter two choices, as the heavy Wyoming snow made three- or four-hour bus trips even longer or often impossible.

Typical of the schools Miner visited was a one-room building with electricity and a butane gas heater. The students in the ten schools in the northern part of the county numbered from one to seven, and all were within bicycle or horseback distance. A hot noonday meal was obtained at the nearest house, or the children brought their own lunch if the distance was too far. As for the teacher, she lived in a room adjoining the schoolhouse, or in the schoolroom itself, as was the case in a trailer-schoolhouse-home. The teacher could leave the building and travel what was probably at least thirty miles to town if she wanted; but once winter came, the blizzards held her captive.

At a school with five students, the teacher seemed concerned over a child with a heart murmur, another with hay fever, and two with poor eating habits. The nurse suggested that the teacher talk to the parents about the first two, feeling that the teacher would know the family better than the nurse. For the problem eaters, teaching material was left with the teacher, who hoped to stress nutrition via a gardening project.

Behavior problems were a concern to some teachers, and Miner would be consulted. One teacher was worried over the play patterns of three of her four students. They played with dump trucks – always in the same pattern, picking the rocks up in a certain spot, dragging the trucks on a beaten path, and then unloading and reloading the rocks. The teacher feared they were not getting enough outside stimuli, and Miner suggested using some audiovisual aids which the teacher agreed to, providing she could find a projector.

At another school, Miner might be invited to eat lunch with a family and observe habits, such as that of a boy whose mother was concerned with his "food jags" where he subsisted on only bread, potatoes, jam, and butter. In this case she decided the "jags" were an attention-getting device that he would outgrow, and suggested that the mother try as best she could to supplement his diet when he was on the "jags."

Most children Miner saw were in exceptionally good health, however. When families live so far from physicians and hospitals, they often have to learn how to take care of themselves, and there is a push on preventive medicine, said Miner, citing that immunization levels of ranch children are often higher than those in urban Wyoming. "However, most of the 31 children with whom I came in contact [in the Laramie Peak area] had not been exposed to the usual childhood diseases such as chicken pox, measles, and mumps, and probably won't be until they reach high school age.

"The time I spent visiting these schools – Antelope Creek, Cozy Hollow, Cottonwood and the rest – was interesting and rewarding," said Miner. "The greatest rewards are the proud looks on parents' faces when they are complimented on their children's obvious good health and the feeling of accomplishment when one learns that health recommendations made the previous year have been carried out – progress in spite of isolation."

Selected References

Bargen, J. Arnold, M.D. "A Community Medical Assistance Plan." *Minnesota Medicine* (January 1959).

Crockett, F. S., M.D. "Looking Back to Look Ahead in Rural Health." *Public Health Reports* (May 1953), vol. 68, no. 5.

Davis, Norman H. "More Doctors in Small Communities." *GP* (March 1958), vol. XVII, no. 3.

"Doctors Up to Date." *Newsweek* (March 22, 1954), vol. 43.

Furlong, William Barry. "Vanishing American – The Country Doctor." New York *Times*, September 7, 1958.

Kane, Robert L.; *et al.* "Mail Order Medicine: An Analysis of the Sears Roebuck Foundation's Community Medical Assistance Program." Salt Lake City: University of Utah, Department of Family and Community Medicine. 1973. Unpublished manuscript.

Kauvar, S. S., M.D.; *et al.* "Health – Twenty Years Late." *American Journal of Public Health* (February 1950), vol. 40.

Maisel, Albert Q. "Dr. Sabin's Second Career." *Survey Graphic* (February 1947), vol. 36.

"Medical Missionaries." *Newsweek* (February 16, 1953), vol. 41.

Michaelson, Mike. "Wyoming's War on Deadly Strep." *Today's Health* (March 1971), vol. 49.

Miner, Jan. "Wyoming School Nurse." *American Journal of Nursing* (September 1965), vol. 65, no. 9.

Moser, Glenda J. "The Quest for Rural Medical Care." *GP* (January 1954), vol. 31, no. 1.

"National Conference on Rural Health." *Journal of the American Medical Association* (June 8, 1946), vol. 131, no. 6.

Sabin, Florence R., M.D. "The People Win for Public Health in Colorado." *American Journal of Public Health* (October 1947), vol. 37.

U.S. Department of Health, Education, and Welfare. *The Economic and Social Condition of Rural America in the 1970s: Impact of Department of HEW Programs on Nonmetropolitan Areas, Fiscal 1970.* Washington, D.C.: U.S. Government Printing Office. 1971.

______________. "Facts about the Hill-Burton Program, July 1, 1947–June 30, 1973." Leaflet of the Office of Planning and Analysis. Rockville, Maryland. No date.

Utah State Medical Association. *Handbook for Delegates.* Salt Lake City: Utah State Medical Association. September 4 and 5, 1957.

7

A Statistical Overview of Health in the Intermountain West

Not until the end of World War II did rural health and health care become recognized as a serious problem common throughout the nation and one which should be dealt with in an organized, systematic way. Large organizations such as the AMA and the Sears, Roebuck Foundation had begun experimenting with programs for improved rural health. Crusading individuals such as Colorado's Florence Sabin became involved. Medical schools began addressing themselves to the problem. Articles on rural health delivery problems were printed profusely in medical journals and other magazines. It was a subject of much discussion and scientific analysis. The importance of social and economic characteristics to the issue of good health came to be recognized. Population and income levels were studied and compared. Reliable statistical data became a crucial element in planning and providing improved health care for rural residents.

This chapter, statistically oriented, is intended to provide the reader with a clear picture of rural health care development and its current status in the Intermountain Region. While the data are not comprehensive or entirely current, they do provide the most thorough and up-to-date record available at the time research and compilation were undertaken for this book.

Rural Population Trends

For the past five decades, the rural population of the United States (defined by the Census Bureau as those living in areas of 2,500 or less population) has remained fairly steady at about fifty million, while the urban population has grown from 54 million to 149 million. In the decade from 1960 to 1970 alone, the urban population grew 19.2 percent, with the rural population declining 0.3 percent.

During the same period, the rural population has become increasingly nonfarm. Three-fifths of the rural population lived on farms in 1920. By 1970, this was down to one-fifth. The nation now has less than ten million people living on farms – only 4.8 percent of the total population.

The Intermountain Region is following the national trend toward decreasing rural population. From 1960 to 1970, as shown in Table 7–1, the rural population in the Intermountain West generally decreased, while the suburban areas outside the central cities, in which the standard metropolitan statistical areas (SMSAS) are concentrated, greatly increased in population.[1] The percentage of rural residents living on farms has also decreased (Table 7–2). However, the states in the Intermountain Area are still somewhat more rural than the United States as a whole (Table 7–3).

In 1970 in the Intermountain Region, 28.3 percent of the residents lived in rural areas, ranging from 19.1 percent in Nevada to 46.6 percent in Montana. Many people continue to be non-city residents, preferring to live in a rural rather than an urban environment. From 1971 to 1972, for the first time in fifty years, more people nationwide migrated *to* instead of *from* farms. The net migration was 150,000 persons, not enough to change the percentage of rural population figures for the nation but nevertheless indicative of a change in migration patterns.

It may be that the comparative advantages of living in a small, local economy are not only attractive to the farm-oriented families and those wishing to live far from the hubbub and turmoil of the city, but also to industry and commercial businesses. Indeed,

[1]The SMSAS, broadly defined, are those areas with a central city of fifty thousand or more population and adjoining areas, sometimes the entire county in which the city is located, sometimes also neighboring counties or parts of counties whose economic and social interests are integrated with the central city/county.

Table 7-1

Percentage of Change in Rural, Urban, and Metropolitan Populations in the Intermountain West (1960–70)

Intermountain State	Percentage of Population Change		
	Urban	Rural	Suburban[a]
Colorado	+34.1%	+ 2.8%	+ 55.5%
Idaho	+21.6	− 6.6	(b)
Montana	+ 9.5	− 3.7	+ 7.4
Nevada	+97.0	+10.4	+104.1
Utah	+27.6	− 7.0	+ 73.5
Wyoming	+ 7.2	− 7.9	(b)
All states	+31.1	− 2.6	+ 57.5

[a]Outside the central cities.

[b]No 1960 standard metropolitan statistical areas (SMSAs). Since this is the SMSA category, there is no basis for comparison.

Source: Bureau of the Census, U.S. Department of Commerce, **Census of the Population, 1970** (Washington, D.C.: U.S. Government Printing Office, 1973).

many of the latter two have located in rural communities, both to their advantage and to that of the residents. But for those people living in rural areas, many factors basic to why they chose to live there in the first place are the very elements which make good health care — and its attendant need of trained personnel and adequate facilities — difficult to obtain.

Problems Confronting Rural Populations

Sparsity of Inhabitants. Rural areas, by nature and by definition, have small populations on large ranches and farms — scattered families who live far from a city's health care facilities. Few states in the Union can claim the sparsity of population that is inherent in the Intermountain West, however, for it is in those states which straddle the Rocky Mountains that several counties average one person per square mile (Table 7–4); some are categorized by the government as "less than one person per square mile" (U.S. Department of Health, Education, and Welfare, 1971). For

Table 7-2

Percentage of Rural Farm and Nonfarm Families in the Intermountain Region and the United States (1960 and 1970)

State or Area	1960		1970	
	Farm	Nonfarm	Farm	Nonfarm
Colorado	28.3%	71.7%	19.1%	80.9%
Idaho	38.0	62.0	29.1	70.9
Montana	32.0	68.0	26.2	73.8
Nevada	12.4	87.6	7.8	92.2
Utah	18.7	81.3	12.6	87.4
Wyoming	30.3	69.7	24.5	75.5
All states Intermountain Region	29.3	70.7	21.6	78.4
United States	25.3	74.7	16.0	84.0

Source: Bureau of the Census, U.S. Department of Commerce, **Census of the Population, 1960** (Washington, D.C.: U.S. Government Printing Office, 1963); Bureau of the Census, U.S. Department of Commerce, **Census of the Population, 1970** (Washington, D.C.: U.S. Government Printing Office, 1973).

example, Nevada has two cities with a population of more than 25,000 and only five cities with more than a thousand residents. In Montana, Idaho, and Wyoming, 45 percent of the population live in communities of 2,500 or less. Utah and Colorado each has the majority of its residents in several urban areas, with the remainder scattered across the rest of the state.

Wherever there is sparse population, there is often a shortage of physicians. Long-standing statistics give vivid testimony to the general movement of physicians away from the rural communities, creating serious gaps in the availability of primary care service. In Colorado, for example, according to Mueller's report (1971), "The geographic distribution of physicians is very uneven for the state, and the gulf between the rural and urban regions is widening." This report also tells us that half of the state's twelve planning districts that existed in 1971 (there are now thirteen such districts) have had substantial decreases in their physician-population ratios within the last seven years, and in 1970 there were four rural counties in Colorado with no doctor whatsoever.

Table 7-3

Average Population in Urban and Rural, Metropolitan and Nonmetropolitan Areas in the Intermountain Region (1970)

State or Area	Total Population	Urban	Rural		Metropolitan	Nonmetroplolitan	
			Number	Percent		Number	Percent
Colorado	2,207,259	1,733,311	473,948	21.5%	1,581,739	625,520	28.3%
Idaho	712,567	385,434	327,133	45.6	112,230	600,337	84.2
Montana	694,409	370,676	323,733	46.6	169,171	525,238	75.6
Nevada	488,738	395,336	93,402	19.1	394,356	94,382	19.3
Utah	1,059,273	851,472	207,801	19.6	821,689	237,584	22.4
Wyoming[a]	332,416	201,111	131,305	39.5	(a)	332,416	100.0
All states in Intermountain Region	5,494,662	3,937,340	1,557,322	28.3[b]	3,079,185	2,415,477	44.0[c]

[a]Wyoming had no SMSAs in 1970.

[b]Percentage for the United States was 26.5 in 1970.

[c]Percentage for the United States was 31.4 in 1970.

Source: Bureau of the Census, U.S. Department of Commerce, **Census of the Housing, 1970** (Washington, D.C.: U.S. Government Printing Office, 1972).

Table 7-4

Rurality of the Population
(1970)

State and County	Total Population (in thousands)	Percent Rural	Population per Square Mile
Colorado:			
Adams	185.9	6.3%	149
Alamosa	11.4	39.4	16
Arapahoe	162.0	2.5	199
Archuleta	2.7	100.0	2
Baca	5.6	100.0	2
Bent	6.4	50.0	4
Boulder	131.8	22.1	176
Chaffee	10.1	57.4	10
Cheyenne	2.4	100.0	1
Clear Creek	4.8	100.0	12
Conejos	7.8	100.0	6
Costilla	3.0	100.0	2
Crowley	3.0	100.0	4
Custer	1.1	100.0	1
Delta	15.2	75.6	13
Denver	514.7	0.0	7,569
Dolores	1.7	100.0	2
Douglas	8.3	100.0	10
Eagle	7.5	100.0	4
Elbert	3.9	100.0	2
El Paso	235.9	11.4	109
Fremont	22.0	32.2	14
Garfield	14.8	72.2	5
Gilpin	1.3	100.0	9
Grand	4.1	100.0	2
Gunnison	7.5	36.0	2
Hinsdale	0.2	100.0	(a)
Huerfano	6.5	29.2	4
Jackson	1.8	100.0	1
Jefferson	233.0	10.1	297
Kiowa	2.0	100.0	1
Kit Carson	7.5	61.3	3
Lake	8.2	47.5	22
La Plata	19.2	44.2	11
Larimer	89.9	33.7	34
Las Animas	15.8	37.3	3

[a] Less than one person per square mile.

Table 7-4 (continued)

State and County	Total Population (in thousands)	Percent Rural	Population per Square Mile
Colorado (continued)			
Lincoln	4.8	100.0	2
Logan	18.8	42.5	10
Mesa	54.3	52.1	16
Mineral	0.8	100.0	1
Moffat	6.5	33.8	1
Montezuma	12.9	51.9	6
Montrose	18.4	64.6	8
Morgan	20.0	45.0	16
Otero	23.4	45.2	19
Ouray	1.5	100.0	3
Park	2.2	100.0	1
Phillips	4.1	100.0	6
Pitkin	6.1	100.0	6
Prowers	13.2	40.9	8
Pueblo	118.3	12.4	49
Rio Blanco	4.8	100.0	1
Rio Grande	10.4	62.5	11
Routt	6.6	100.0	3
Saguache	3.8	100.0	1
San Juan	0.8	100.0	2
San Miguel	1.9	100.0	1
Sedgwick	3.4	100.0	6
Summit	2.7	100.0	4
Teller	3.3	100.0	6
Washington	5.5	100.0	2
Weld	89.3	53.5	22
Yuma	8.5	100.0	4
Idaho:			
Ada	112.3	21.9	108
Adams	2.9	100.0	2
Bannock	52.1	17.2	46
Bear Lake	5.8	53.4	6
Benewah	6.2	59.6	8
Bingham	29.2	61.3	14
Blaine	5.7	100.0	2
Boise	1.7	100.0	1
Bonner	15.5	72.9	9
Bonneville	51.2	30.0	28
Boundary	6.4	56.2	5
Butte	2.9	100.0	1

Table 7-4 (continued)

State and County	Total Population (in thousands)	Percent Rural	Population per Square Mile
Idaho (continued)			
Camas	0.7	100.0	1
Canyon	61.3	42.9	106
Caribou	6.5	53.8	4
Cassia	17.0	52.3	7
Clark	0.7	100.0	(a)
Clearwater	10.8	63.8	4
Custer	2.9	100.0	1
Elmore	17.5	28.0	6
Franklin	7.3	53.4	11
Fremont	8.7	67.8	5
Gem	9.3	58.0	17
Gooding	8.6	69.7	12
Idaho	12.9	71.3	2
Jefferson	11.6	100.0	11
Jerome	10.2	57.8	17
Kootenai	35.3	54.1	28
Latah	24.9	43.3	23
Lemhi	5.5	47.2	1
Lewis	3.9	100.0	8
Lincoln	3.0	100.0	2
Madison	13.4	35.0	28
Minidoka	15.8	70.2	21
Nez Perce	30.3	13.8	36
Oneida	2.9	100.0	2
Owyhee	6.4	100.0	1
Payette	12.4	62.9	31
Power	4.8	33.3	3
Shoshone	19.7	79.1	8
Teton	2.3	100.0	5
Twin Falls	41.9	40.5	22
Valley	3.6	100.0	1
Washington	7.6	42.1	5
Montana:			
Beaverhead	8.1	43.2	1
Big Horn	10.0	73.0	2
Blaine	6.7	100.0	2
Broadwater	2.5	100.0	2
Carbon	7.0	100.0	3

[a] Less than one person per square mile.

Table 7-4 (continued)

State and County	Total Population (in thousands)	Percent Rural	Population per Square Mile
Montana (continued)			
Carter	1.9	100.0	1
Cascade	81.9	13.3	31
Chouteau	6.5	100.0	2
Custer	12.2	26.2	3
Daniels	3.1	100.0	2
Dawson	11.3	41.5	5
Deer Lodge	15.5	36.7	21
Fallon	4.0	30.0	2
Fergus	12.6	46.8	3
Flathead	39.4	58.1	8
Gallatin	32.5	42.4	13
Garfield	1.8	100.0	(a)
Glacier	10.8	62.9	4
Golden Valley	0.9	100.0	1
Granite	2.7	100.0	2
Hill	17.4	39.6	6
Jefferson	5.3	100.0	3
Judith Basin	2.7	100.0	1
Lake	14.4	100.0	10
Lewis and Clark	33.3	31.8	10
Liberty	2.3	100.0	2
Lincoln	18.0	81.6	5
Madison	5.0	100.0	1
McCone	2.9	100.0	1
Meagher	2.1	100.0	1
Mineral	2.9	100.0	2
Missoula	58.3	25.5	22
Musselshell	3.7	100.0	2
Park	11.1	36.0	4
Petroleum	0.7	100.0	(a)
Phillips	5.4	100.0	1
Pondera	6.6	53.0	4
Powder River	2.8	100.0	1
Powell	6.6	31.8	3
Prairie	1.7	100.0	1
Ravalli	14.3	100.0	6
Richland	9.8	53.0	5
Roosevelt	10.3	69.9	4
Rosebud	6.0	100.0	1

[a] Less than one person per square mile.

Table 7-4 (continued)

State and County	Total Population (in thousands)	Percent Rural	Population per Square Mile
Montana (continued)			
Sanders	7.1	100.0	3
Sheridan	5.7	100.0	3
Silver Bow	42.1	19.0	59
Stillwater	4.6	100.0	3
Sweet Grass	3.0	100.0	2
Teton	6.1	100.0	3
Toole	5.9	47.4	3
Treasure	1.1	100.0	1
Valley	11.5	59.1	2
Wheatland	2.5	100.0	2
Wibaux	1.5	100.0	2
Yellowstone	87.4	13.5	33
Nevada:			
Churchill	10.4	71.1	2
Clark	273.2	5.4	35
Douglas	6.8	100.0	9
Elko	13.9	45.0	1
Esmeralda	0.6	100.0	(a)
Eureka	0.9	100.0	(a)
Humboldt	6.3	42.8	1
Lander	2.6	100.0	(a)
Lincoln	2.6	100.0	(a)
Lyon	8.2	100.0	4
Mineral	7.0	50.0	2
Nye	5.5	100.0	(a)
Pershing	2.6	100.0	(a)
Storey	0.7	100.0	3
Washoe	121.0	17.6	19
White Pine	10.1	58.4	1
Ormsby	15.4	0.6	109
Utah:			
Beaver	3.8	100.0	1
Box Elder	28.2	40.4	5
Cache	42.4	39.1	36
Carbon	15.6	59.6	11
Daggett	0.6	100.0	1
Davis	99.0	13.7	333

[a]Less than one person per square mile.

Table 7-4 (continued)

State and County	Total Population (in thousands)	Percent Rural	Population per Square Mile
Utah (continued)			
Duchesne	7.2	100.0	2
Emery	5.1	100.0	1
Garfield	3.1	100.0	1
Grand	6.6	22.7	2
Iron	12.2	25.4	4
Juab	4.5	33.3	1
Kane	2.4	100.0	1
Millard	7.0	100.0	1
Morgan	4.0	100.0	7
Piute	1.1	100.0	1
Rich	1.6	100.0	2
Salt Lake	458.6	4.8	600
San Juan	9.5	100.0	1
Sanpete	10.9	100.0	7
Sevier	10.1	54.4	5
Summit	5.9	100.0	3
Tooele	21.5	28.3	3
Uintah	12.6	67.4	3
Utah	137.7	12.3	68
Wasatch	5.8	44.8	5
Washington	13.7	48.1	6
Wayne	1.5	100.0	1
Weber	126.2	12.5	217
Wyoming:			
Albany	26.4	12.8	6
Big Horn	10.1	100.0	3
Campbell	12.9	44.1	3
Carbon	13.3	40.6	2
Converse	5.9	59.3	1
Crook	4.5	100.0	2
Fremont	28.3	46.6	3
Goshen	10.8	61.1	5
Hot Springs	4.9	36.7	2
Johnson	5.6	37.5	1
Laramie	56.3	19.5	21
Lincoln	8.6	100.0	2
Natrona	51.2	22.8	10
Niobrara	2.9	100.0	1
Park	17.9	44.6	3
Platte	6.4	100.0	3

Table 7-4 (continued)

State and County	Total Population (in thousands)	Percent Rural	Population per Square Mile
Wyoming (continued)			
Sheridan	17.8	38.7	7
Sublette	3.7	100.0	1
Sweetwater	18.2	12.0	2
Teton	4.8	100.0	1
Uinta	7.0	37.1	3
Washakie	7.4	31.0	3
Weston	NA	NA	NA

NA = not available.

Source: Bureau of Health Resources, Divison of Manpower Intelligence, U.S. Department of Health, Education, and Welfare, **Area Resource File** (Rockville, Maryland, April 1974).

Some of these Colorado areas have not had doctors for years, or possibly have had from one to five doctors who move on after a brief stay, says Dr. Monroe Tyler,[2] who has long served on Colorado's Rural Health Committee and was formerly a member of the American Medical Association's Council on Rural Health. "These areas are the same today as they were many years ago. My feeling is that these areas will never have a doctor who will be permanent."

In Nevada, Comprehensive Health Planning Coordinator Herb Pevney[3] says that the state's more populous counties (Clark and Washoe) have one doctor for every 1,045 and 555 persons respectively (1972 data), while the remaining fourteen and less populous counties have one physician for every 1,681 persons.

Wyoming, Montana, Nevada, and Idaho are by numerous definitions "medically underserved," says Erickson (1972). In 1969, the national ratio of physicians per hundred thousand population was 163; within the four-state area, the rate was 105. And rural Utah faces many of these same problems.

Misleading Rates. Table 7–5 lists the number of physicians by county and gives physician-population ratios. But one must beware when studying such data. "In addition to whole counties, there are

[2]Correspondence, March 6, 1975, now in the files of the authors.

[3]Telephone interview, March 26, 1975.

Table 7-5

Ratios of Active Physicians to Population in the Intermountain West[a]
(1971 and 1972)

State, County, and Type of Area	Total Number of Physicians	Rate per Thousand Population
Colorado:		
Rural		
Archuleta	1	0.37
Baca	4	0.71
Cheyenne	2	0.84
Clear Creek	2	0.42
Conejos	5	0.64
Costilla	1	0.33
Crowley	2	0.66
Custer	0	
Dolores	0	
Douglas	8	0.96
Eagle	3	0.40
Elbert	0	
Gilpin	1	0.77
Grand	3	0.73
Hinsdale	0	
Jackson	1	0.56
Kiowa	1	0.50
Lincoln	2	0.42
Mineral	0	
Ouray	1	0.67
Park	1	0.45
Phillips	3	0.73
Pitkin	19	3.11
Rio Blanco	4	0.83
Routt	7	1.06
Saguache	2	0.53
San Juan	1	1.25
San Miguel	2	1.06
Sedgwick	2	0.59
Summit	2	0.74
Teller	2	0.61
Washington	1	0.18
Yuma	4	0.47

[a]Includes 1972 M.D.s and 1971 D.O.s.

Table 7-5 (continued)

State, County, and Type of Area	Total Number of Physicians	Rate per Thousand Population
Colorado (continued)		
Predominantly rural		
Bent	2	0.31
Chaffee	9	0.89
Delta	9	0.60
Garfield	16	1.08
Kit Carson	2	0.27
Mesa	93	1.72
Montezuma	9	0.70
Montrose	16	0.87
Rio Grande	9	0.87
Weld	103	1.15
Predominantly urban		
Adams	104	0.56
Alamosa	14	1.23
Arapahoe	218	1.35
Boulder	210	1.60
Denver	2,308	4.49
El Paso	280	1.19
Fremont	20	0.91
Gunnison	4	0.53
Huerfano	4	0.62
Jefferson	205	0.88
Lake	7	0.85
La Plata	34	1.77
Larimer	118	1.32
Las Animas	6	0.38
Logan	20	1.07
Moffat	5	0.77
Morgan	12	0.60
Otero	19	0.81
Prowers	7	0.53
Pueblo	155	1.31
Idaho:		
Rural		
Adams	1	0.34
Blaine	9	1.58
Boise	0	
Butte	2	0.69
Camas	1	1.43
Clark	0	

Table 7-5 (continued)

State, County, and Type of Area	Total Number of Physicians	Rate per Thousand Population
Idaho (continued)		
Custer	0	
Jefferson	3	0.26
Lewis	3	0.77
Lincoln	1	0.33
Oneida	1	0.34
Owyhee	0	
Teton	1	0.43
Valley	7	1.95
Predominantly rural		
Bear Lake	4	0.69
Benewah	4	0.65
Bingham	13	0.44
Bonner	11	0.71
Boundary	3	0.47
Caribou	3	0.46
Cassia	13	0.76
Clearwater	6	0.56
Franklin	3	0.41
Fremont	5	0.57
Gem	4	0.43
Gooding	7	0.81
Idaho	9	0.70
Jerome	7	0.69
Kootenai	40	1.13
Minidoka	7	0.44
Payette	4	0.32
Shoshone	11	0.56
Predominantly urban		
Ada	171	1.52
Bannock	61	1.17
Bonneville	62	1.21
Canyon	75	1.23
Elmore	8	0.46
Latah	23	0.92
Lemhi	5	0.91
Madison	7	0.52
Nez Perce	48	1.59
Power	3	0.63
Twin Falls	63	1.50
Washington	3	0.39

Table 7-5 (continued)

State, County, and Type of Area	Total Number of Physicians	Rate per Thousand Population
Montana:		
Rural		
Blaine	4	0.60
Broadwater	3	1.20
Carbon	4	0.57
Carter	1	0.53
Chouteau	2	0.31
Daniels	2	0.65
Garfield	1	0.56
Golden Valley	0	
Granite	1	0.37
Jefferson	1	0.19
Judith Basin	0	
Lake	11	0.76
Liberty	1	0.43
Madison	5	1.00
McCone	1	0.34
Meagher	1	0.43
Mineral	1	0.34
Musselshell	2	0.54
Petroleum	0	
Phillips	2	0.37
Powder River	1	0.36
Prairie	0	
Ravalli	10	0.70
Rosebud	3	0.50
Sanders	5	0.70
Sheridan	2	0.35
Stillwater	2	0.43
Sweet Grass	2	0.67
Teton	3	0.49
Treasure	0	
Wheatland	2	0.80
Wibaux	0	
Predominantly rural		
Big Horn	2	0.20
Flathead	53	1.35
Glacier	5	0.46
Lincoln	8	0.44
Pondera	4	0.61
Richland	6	0.61

Table 7-5 (continued)

State, County, and Type of Area	Total Number of Physicians	Rate per Thousand Population
Montana (continued)		
Roosevelt	6	0.58
Valley	5	0.43
Predominantly urban		
Beaverhead	4	0.49
Cascade	100	1.22
Custer	18	1.48
Dawson	8	0.71
Deer Lodge	21	1.35
Fallon	2	0.50
Fergus	6	0.48
Gallatin	45	1.38
Hill	13	0.75
Lewis and Clark	51	1.53
Missoula	102	1.75
Park	12	1.08
Powell	9	1.36
Silver Bow	47	1.11
Toole	3	0.51
Yellowstone	134	1.59
Nevada:		
Rural		
Douglas	5	0.74
Esmeralda	0	
Eureka	1	1.11
Lander	1	0.38
Lincoln	1	0.38
Lyon	3	0.37
Nye	2	0.36
Pershing	3	1.15
Storey	0	
Predominantly rural		
Churchill	4	0.38
Mineral	2	0.29
White Pine	6	0.59
Predominantly urban		
Clark	277	1.01
Elko	14	1.01

Table 7-5 (continued)

State, County, and Type of Area	Total Number of Physicians	Rate per Thousand Population
Nevada (continued)		
Humboldt	3	0.48
Washoe	227	1.87
Ormsby	25	1.62
Utah:		
Rural		
Beaver	3	0.79
Daggett	0	
Duchesne	4	0.56
Emery	2	0.39
Garfield	1	0.32
Kane	3	1.25
Millard	5	0.71
Morgan	3	0.75
Piute	0	
Rich	0	
San Juan	5	0.53
Sanpete	7	0.64
Summit	3	0.51
Wayne	0	
More than 50 percent rural		
Carbon	13	0.83
Sevier	6	0.59
Uintah	5	0.40
Predominantly urban		
Box Elder	16	0.57
Cache	42	0.99
Davis	49	0.49
Grand	5	0.76
Iron	10	0.82
Juab	3	0.67
Salt Lake	1,085	2.36
Tooele	10	0.47
Utah	129	0.94
Wasatch	4	0.69
Washington	10	0.73
Weber	164	1.30
Wyoming:		
Rural		
Big Horn	6	0.59

Table 7-5 (continued)

State, County, and Type of Area	Total Number of Physicians	Rate per Thousand Population
Wyoming (continued)		
Crook	2	0.44
Lincoln	5	0.58
Niobrara	1	0.34
Platte	3	0.47
Sublette	2	0.54
Teton	11	2.29
Predominantly rural		
Converse	4	0.68
Goshen	9	0.83
Weston	NA	NA
Predominantly urban		
Albany	24	0.91
Campbell	5	0.39
Carbon	13	0.98
Fremont	27	0.95
Hot Springs	4	0.82
Johnson	5	0.89
Laramie	71	1.26
Natrona	63	1.23
Park	15	0.84
Sheridan	22	1.24
Sweetwater	14	0.77
Uinta	11	1.57
Washakie	8	1.08

NA = Not available.

Source: Bureau of Health Resources, Division of Manpower Intelligence, U.S. Department of Health, Education, and Welfare, **Area Resource File** (Rockville, Maryland, April 1974).

towns within counties which cannot support a physician and are extremely far from medical services," reads the *Montana State Plan for Health* (Montana State, 1974):

> ... For example, Fergus County has a physician-population ratio of 1 to 1,576, but all doctors are located in Lewistown. Towns like Denton, population 398, which is 39 miles away over mainly secondary roads, and Winifred, population 220,

> which is 38 miles away, cannot support a physician. The fact is that even where there is a physician available "statistically" in some of Montana's larger but less populous counties, it is a physical impossibility for the physician to service the large areas. He cannot get to the people and they cannot get to him. In addition, while much of Montana surpasses most of the rest of the U.S. in recreational opportunities and sheer esthetic appeal, there are portions of the state which do not have these features. Coupled with this, small numbers of people cannot support man-made amenities (e.g., cultural and educational opportunities) to the extent necessary to attract professional people.

There are other ways in which doctor-patient ratios can be misleading. Utah's Wasatch Front, which includes Salt Lake City, has a much higher physician-patient ratio than the remainder of the state. In fact, at first glance (see Table 7–5) the area almost appears to be oversaturated with doctors. Yet, according to *Utah Health Facts* (Utah State, 1972):

> . . . [In] proportion to the large population in the Front, there does not appear to be an oversupply. When the analysis is refined with the intent to exclude nonpracticing physicians and specialists (by switching from licensed physicians to AAMPC [advertised available primary medical care] physicians), the rate per 1,000 residents in the Front is not strikingly different from the rates in the more rural counties (except for the four counties with no physician).

In Colorado, according to Mueller's survey (1971), which quotes Frank Dickeson, former director of the AMA's Bureau of Medical Economics, "The population-physician ratio . . . reminds one of attempts to measure supply and demand by county buyers and sellers." Mueller himself continues:

> Unless demand for health services is directly proportional to population and, simultaneously, supply of health services is directly proportional to the numbers of available members in a health manpower category, these ratios are not very accurate indicators of the true demand for and supply of health care services. Demand for health services depends upon a number of socioeconomic factors, among which are: consumer income, prices of health services, prices of other goods and services, education, etc. Similarly, the supply of health services depends

upon a number of variables in addition to the number of available health manpower resources.

Consumer Income. When one of these factors, consumer income, is low and the area is a sparsely populated one, physician manpower ratios and other health statistics can resemble those of an undeveloped nation. And while the scenic Intermountain West may not resemble struggling African countries, rural incomes in the Mountain states are consistently lower than the urban incomes and are often below or near the national averages, which include the incomes of the poor in the South and in Appalachia.

Health care costs are rising at a rapid pace and are not expected to decline in the near future. This magnifies the problem of the rural poor who, although they pay less than city dwellers, spend a larger percentage of their income for medical care. From 1950 to 1971, total health expenditures rose from $12 billion to $75 billion (U.S. Department of Agriculture, 1973). As a percentage of the gross national product, they went from 4.6 to 7.4. For each American, these large expenditures meant an average 1971 health bill of $358, more than two and a half times the bill of 1960, and four and a half times that of 1950. Early estimates of the 1980 health care costs, made before the rapid rise of inflation of the 1970s, was $814 per person, according to the Department of Agriculture. During the 1962–72 decade, claims DuVal (1972), Assistant Secretary for Health and Scientific Affairs at the Department of Health, Education, and Welfare, 60 percent of the increase went to meet the cost of inflation, not to pay for better or more health care.

As costs continue to climb because of inflation, rural residents will pay an increasingly higher percentage of their incomes for medical care. In the past forty years, per capita income in nonmetropolitan areas has been rising at a faster rate than that of metropolitan areas, but the percentage gain has not been fast enough to narrow the gap between metropolitan and nonmetropolitan incomes. Instead, the dollar difference has widened over the years. Nonmetropolitan personal income, which increased at an average rate of 7.4 percent per year, compared with 5.9 percent for metropolitan areas, would have had to grow at the rate of 8.5 percent for this forty-year period to have closed the gap.

However, for all of the western states from Colorado to California, Oregon, and Washington, there is a continued lag in nonmetropolitan income growth. The fast acceleration of national nonmetropolitan income growth was in the Plains states, where recovery from low nonmetropolitan farm income in 1959 and large gains in manufacturing made the difference (U.S. Congress, 1971).

In Table 7–6, family incomes are divided into categories of rural farm, rural nonfarm, and "other" urban or suburban. In 1970, the lowest average income for the Intermountain Region was that of rural farm families, with the mean being $9,149. Rural nonfarm incomes averaged $9,373 for the area. Both of these figures were higher than the national averages of $8,677 and $9,184 respectively, but were considerably lower than the mean suburban figure for the Intermountain Area. Mean income for suburban residents in the United States was $13,271, and all suburban incomes for the Intermountain West were more than $11,000, except Montana, which had a mean suburban income of $8,569, lower than its mean farm income.

Rural family income is generally lower than other mean family incomes, and a greater proportion of rural people live below the national poverty line. Nearly twice as many Americans below the poverty level, as defined by the Census Bureau in 1969, were from nonmetropolitan areas as compared to metropolitan areas. The number of farm families below the poverty level is consistently higher than that for nonfarm families (U.S. Congress, 1971). Poverty in rural America dominates the lives of twelve million (17 percent) of the rural population. One out of every six persons in rural areas lives in poverty, as compared with one out of ten in urban areas (U.S. Department of Agriculture, 1973).

In the Intermountain Region, only Nevada is consistently above the national median of poverty for both rural and urban residents (Table 7–7). All of the six states' urban areas have a smaller percentage of poverty-level families than the rural areas. In Wyoming, 8.3 percent of the urban residents are low income, while 12.5 percent of the rural farm residents fit in this category. The figures for Montana are 8.2 percent for urbanites and 14.5 percent for farm residents; for Utah, they are 8.4 percent for urban and 12.7 percent for farm families. In all cases, the farm people have the highest rates of poverty, from 9.7 percent in Nevada, whose residents have 6.7 percent of their numbers below the poverty line, to 17 percent of farm people living in Colorado. Nationwide,

Table 7-6

Mean and Median Income Levels in the Intermountain Region, by Rural Farm, Rural Nonfarm, and Urban or Suburban Families

(1970)

State or Area	Rural Farm Income		Rural Nonfarm Income		Other Urban of Suburban Income	
	Median	Mean	Median	Mean	Median	Mean
Colorado	$7,103	$8,632	$8,421	$9,667	$11,164	$12,366
Idaho	7,584	9,078	8,018	8,800	10,138	11,099
Montana	7,367	9,369	8,052	8,813	7,957	8,569
Nevada	8,921	12,484	10,023	11,141	10,551	11,600
Utah	7,898	9,073	8,261	8,845	10,389	11,391
Wyoming	7,506	9,551	8,486	9,339	—	—
All states in Intermountain Region		9,149		9,373		12,049
United States	7,082	8,677	8,231	9,184	11,586	13,271

Source: Bureau of the Census, U.S. Department of Commerce, **Census of the Population, 1970** (Washington, D.C.: U.S. Government Printing Office, 1973).

Table 7-7

Families below Poverty Level in the Intermountain States as Compared to the United States Levels[a] (1970)

	Total		Urban Families		Rural Families			
					Nonfarm		Farm	
Variable	Number	Percent	Number	Percent	Number	Percent	Number	Percent
Colorado:								
Families	547,165		425,983		98,078		23,104	
Below poverty line	49,850	9.1%	34,416	8.1%	11,619	11.8%	3,928	17.0%
Idaho:								
Families	179,448		96,828		58,570		24,050	
Below poverty line	19,504	10.9	9,634	9.9	7,002	12.0	2,939	12.2
Montana:								
Families	171,812		91,340		59,411		21,061	
Below poverty line	17,821	10.4	7,503	8.2	7,351	12.4	3,061	14.5
Nevada:								
Families	124,170		100,133		22,180		1,857	
Below poverty line	8,641	7.0	6,650	6.7	1,716	7.7	181	9.7

[a]Rounded to the nearest number.

Table 7-7 (continued)

Variable	Total		Urban Families		Rural Families			
					Nonfarm		Farm	
	Number	Percent	Number	Percent	Number	Percent	Number	Percent
Utah:								
Families	249,741		201,429		42,206		6,106	12.7
Below poverty line	22,802	9.1	16,859	8.4	5,222	12.4	777	
Wyoming:								
Families	84,703		50,764		25,616		8,323	
Below poverty line	7,841	9.3	4,214	8.3	2,613	10.2	1,042	12.5
All states in Intermountain Region:								
Families	1,357,037		966,477		306,061			
Below poverty line	126,459	9.3	79,376	8.2	35,523	11.6	84,501	14.1
United States		10.7		9.0		15.1	11,928	16.4

Source: Bureau of the Census, U.S. Department of Commerce, **Census of the Population, 1970** (Washington, D.C.: U.S. Government Printing Office, 1973).

9 percent of all urban residents are below the poverty line, compared with 16.4 percent of all farm residents.

Low incomes and sparse population prevent rural areas from competing effectively in the medical marketplace; thus deficiencies exist in both the quality and quantity of rurally located medical personnel and facilities. Low incomes also make rural locations unattractive to doctors seeking practice locations. According to Cooper *et al.* (1972):

> One of the chief reasons physicians go into small community practice is the likelihood of developing a busy practice early. Therefore, the economy of the community may be an important determining factor in the choice of location. While studies have shown that there exists a positive relationship between regional per capita income and the supply of physicians, those analyses have usually been done on county or state levels and may not be entirely relevant to the problem of the small communities within these boundaries. However, at least one study has indicated that slow or declining economic growth rates are characteristic of towns without physicians. Also, in another study, the median income of a community's population was significantly higher for towns gaining physicians in a 20-year period than for towns losing physicians. Thus it seems that towns with a low median income or an otherwise poor economy are in an unfavorable position for attracting or retaining physicians.

However, the authors qualify this statement by saying that such a relationship between physician income and physician location is "not as predictable as one might assume."

Other Factors

Specialists. General practitioners are almost evenly distributed throughout the country by population density, but areas of high income and high population density attract more specialists and hospital-based doctors. As a result, rural people do not get the quality of care available to urban residents. Nevada, for example, has no specialists outside its more urban areas of Washoe County (Reno), Clark County (Las Vegas), the city of Elko (in Elko County), and Carson City, according to Herb Pevney. The rest of the state has general practitioners and general surgeons. In the city of Elko, the one specialty doctor is an obstetrician (Elko County is 45 percent rural).

In Colorado in 1970, the statistics on specialists (Table 7–8) paint as grim a picture as those for other Intermountain Area states (Mueller, 1971):

> Of the state's 474 M.D.s practicing outside the three SMSAS, 241 or 51 percent are [general practitioners]. If one looks at the physicians in family care, i.e., GPs, IMs (internists), and PDs (pediatricians) combined, the Denver SMSA and the "rest of the state" area both have more than their proportionate share and the Colorado Springs and Pueblo SMSAS have less. The concentration of the total medical, surgical, and other specialties in the Denver SMSA is very high. The Pueblo SMSA had more specialists per population than the El Paso SMSA; however, both SMSAS fall below their proportionate share. Only in surgical specialties does the Pueblo SMSA exceed its proportionate share. The "rest of the state" lacks in all specialties.

The only specialist found in six of Wyoming's seven most rural counties in 1974 is one gynecologist in Big Horn (Wyoming State, 1974). Teton County is the exception; it has sixteen physicians (as of March 1974), with at least eleven of them being specialists. Within the boundaries of Teton County is Teton National Park, a major outdoor recreational area. In contrast, Wyoming's five most urban counties (Sweetwater, Albany, Laramie, Natrona, and Washakie) have five, 21, 59, 54, and one respectively. Washakie County is 31 percent rural.

Utah's Rich, Piute, Wayne, and Daggett counties, the least densely populated in the state, are entirely rural. Data show that they share in none of the state's total number of specialists; in fact, no resident physicians live in these counties whatsoever (Utah State, 1972).

A lack of specialists in the rural areas can also result in overworked general practitioners who may undertake more complicated surgery and treatment than would the urban general practitioner.

Anesthesiologists. In the 1968 study by Graves *et al.*, the following data concerning anethesiologists in the Intermountain Region buttress this last point. The study showed that the six-state region, which at that time had a population of 5,211,000, had 210 physicians who were members of the American Society of Anesthesiology and 274 active nurse members of the American Association

Table 7-8
Distribution of Nonfederal M.D.s in Colorado, by Specialty of Practice and SMSA
(1970)

Variable	State Total	Standard Metropolitan Statistical Area						Rest of State	
		Denver		Colorado Springs		Pueblo			
		Number	Percent	Number	Percent	Number	Percent	Number	Percent
Population	2,207,259	1,222,529	55.4%	235,972	10.7%	118,238	5.4%	630,520	28.6%
Total M.D.s providing patient care	3,067	2,236	72.9	214	7.0	143	4.7	474	15.4
General practitioner (G.P.)	599	308	51.4	37	6.2	13	2.2	241	40.2
Medical specialties (total)	708	559	78.9	50	7.1	33	4.7	66	9.3
Internal medicine (I.M.)	321	239	74.4	24	7.5	21	6.5	37	11.5
Pediatrics (P.D.)	215	177	82.3	11	5.1	7	3.3	20	9.3
Surgical specialties (total)	908	670	73.8	73	8.0	56	6.2	109	12.0

Table 7-8 (continued)

Variable	State Total	Standard Metropolitan Statistical Area: Denver		Colorado Springs		Pueblo		Rest of State	
		Number	Percent	Number	Percent	Number	Percent	Number	Percent
General surgery (G.S.)	297	214	72.0	17	5.7	18	6.1	48	16.2
Obstetrics-gynecology (O.B.G.)	190	151	79.5	17	8.9	10	5.3	12	6.3
Other specialties	852	699	82.0	54	6.3	41	4.8	58	6.8
Radiology	127	99	77.9	6	4.7	8	6.3	14	11.0
Family Practice (G.P., I.M., P.D.)	1,135	724	63.8	72	6.3	41	3.6	298	26.3

Source: Heinz F. Mueller, M.A., **Colorado Health Consumer Survey — A Regional Analysis: Colorado-Wyoming Regional Medical Program** (Denver: Colorado Office of Comprehensive Health Planning and Colorado-Wyoming Regional Medical Program, May 1971).

of Nurse Anesthesiology. These trained anesthesiologists were located in only 119 communities of the Intermountain West. Moreover, over half of the area's population did not live in areas that had a trained anesthesiologist.

Utah, for example, had the highest ratio of anesthesiologists to total number of physicians in the nation in 1968, but every one of these specialists were located in the Salt Lake City–Ogden–Provo–Logan metropolitan area. All but six of the nurse anesthesiologists were similarly located.

To find out who was administering anesthetics in outlying areas, the Division of Anesthesiology at the University of Utah sent letters to general practitioners in parts of Idaho, Montana, Utah, Nevada, and Wyoming, where surgery and obstetrics were performed, but where no trained anesthesiologists practiced. Among those who replied, 36 percent stated that they themselves administered the anesthetics in their practices, ranging from rarely to regularly. Half of these stated that they had not had special training in anesthesiology. The other half had received some training, usually one to three months during their internship or residency. Only three physicians stated that they had had more than three months' training in administering anesthetics.

Attrition Due to Age. Another rural problem is that of attrition; that is, when the older doctors in the rural areas retire or die, they are not replaced by younger medical graduates. Making this problem worse in the Intermountain Area is the fact that rural doctors are much older than their urban counterparts. Information from the *Wyoming Health Profile* (Wyoming State, 1974) reveals that of the state's seven most rural counties, three have physicians whose average age is over the state mean of 48.7. The three counties are Big Horn (with an average physician age of 52.1 years), Teton (50.7), and Platte (51.3). Crook and Niobrara counties have no ages listed because at that time there were no physicians in those counties; however, National Health Service Corps men were to be assigned to the counties. Lincoln and Sublette counties had doctors whose ages were below the state average at 46 and 45.5 respectively.

Wyoming's more urban counties — Sweetwater (major city, Rock Springs), Albany (Laramie), Laramie County (Cheyenne), Natrona (Casper), and Washakie (Worland) — have doctors whose ages range from 47.8 to 54.8. In the state's 23 counties, the average ages of doctors are as follows:

County and Type of Area	*Average Age of Physicians*
Rural:	
Big Horn	52.1
Crook[4]	
Lincoln	46.0
Niobrara[5]	
Platte	51.3
Sublette	45.5
Teton	50.7
Predominantly rural:	
Converse	46.5
Goshen	49.8
Weston	52.3
Predominantly urban:	
Albany	49.8
Campbell	52.1
Carbon	54.9
Fremont	43.5
Hot Springs	57.6
Johnson	51.5
Laramie	48.8
Natroma	47.9
Park	50.6
Sheridan	51.0
Sweetwater	54.8
Uintah	55.6
Washakie	51.8

Thus we see that ages of doctors in Wyoming are fairly high. This might be a reflection of the general rurality of the entire state: Wyoming's "most urban" county, Fremont, has a population of 18,391. By contrast, Washakie has 7,400 residents and is 31 percent rural.

Not only do rural people generally have older and fewer doctors, they receive visits from their physicians less often then their city counterparts. The western region's average for outside the SMSA is better than the national average, but as can be seen below, when divided into farm and nonfarm categories, the farm inhabitants see their doctors less often, and all western rural people have fewer doctor visits than do western city dwellers. The following

[4]National Health Service Corps physician supplied July 1, 1974, after information was compiled.

[5]National Health Service Corps physicians until July 1975.

shows the number of physician visits per person per year in the United States as compared to the western states (U.S. Department of Health, Education, and Welfare, 1974):

Geographic Variable	*Number of Visits*
United States:	4.4
Standard metropolitan statistical area –	4.6
Central city	4.7
Outside central city	4.5
Large SMSA	4.9
Other SMSA	4.4
Outside SMSA –	4.1
Nonfarm	4.3
Farm	3.2
Western states:	4.8
Standard metropolitan statistical area –	5.0
Central city	5.3
Outside central city	4.7
Large SMSA	5.2
Los Angeles	5.2
San Francisco	5.1
Other SMSA	4.8
Outside SMSA –	4.3
Nonfarm	4.5
Farm	2.9

Income affects how often many people see their doctors, says American Hospital Association President Alex McMahon[6]: "This [low income] not only erects a financial barrier to payment for care, but also discourages care because of the time it takes from necessary farm chores – an additional problem aggravated by the distance barrier."

Nationally, twice as many persons in families with incomes of $7,000 or more, compared with those in families with less than $2,000 annual income, use the services of specialists during a one-year period. In one example (President's National Advisory Commission, 1967), approximately 20 percent of the children under age fifteen were examined or treated by a pediatrician during a one-year period. This proportion was 9.6 percent for those in the lowest

[6]Telephone interview, March 12, 1975.

income groups and 29.4 percent for those families with incomes of \$7,000 or more. Moreover, children in higher income families and those living in metropolitan areas of the country are more likely to have a routine physical examination than those in low income families and those living outside metropolitan areas and especially those on farms. This lack of medical care in the younger years has proved to be tragic because a large portion of the debilitating chronic conditions which handicap youngsters could possibly be prevented or corrected by early detection and proper treatment at appropriate ages in childhood.

The relationship between health care and income is even more striking for dental care (discussed subsequently in detail). The poor rarely see a dentist. A fourth of the poor have never been to a dentist. Only 24 percent of the persons in families with less than \$3,000 annual income, compared with 57 percent of those in families with \$7,000 or more income, visit a dentist during a year (President's National Advisory Commission, 1967).

Expenditures for health care change with income and size of family. A family with \$7,000 or more annual income and three family members spend five times as much on the care of one child as does the seven-member family with an income of \$2,000. In addition, as population density decreases, per capita expenditure also decreases, irrespective of income. According to the President's National Advisory Commission on Rural Poverty, 1967:

> The amount spent on health care is lowest among the low-income rural families and particularly the amount spent for the health care of the very young.... This is consistent with the low level of medical and dental care among rural farm families, as well as the low proportion of persons with health insurance coverage.... Although three-fourths of the people in the United States have some kind of health insurance coverage to protect them against the cost of medical care, unfortunately the poor who need it most do not have such protection. About one-third of the families with income of less than \$2,000 have health insurance, compared with nine-tenths of the persons with income of \$10,000 or more. Regardless of income, the rate of insurance coverage is lowest for rural farm residents, a fact which partially reflects differences in patterns of employment between urban and rural areas. The proportion of persons with insurance protection is lowest for the rural poor on southern farms.

Dentists, Pharmacists, and Auxiliary Health Care Personnel. Lack of money causes other health care problems also. Slow economic growth makes it difficult for towns and small communities to attract physicians and other health care personnel who prefer the higher wages of the city.

The distribution of dentists and pharmacists in Utah is an example of this. According to *Utah Health Facts* (Utah State, 1972), dentists are concentrated along the Wasatch Front counties and absent in several rural ones. Unlike physicians, however, who tend to be located only in the largest communities of a county, dentists are spread into the smaller communities. Pharmacists are also found more frequently in the smaller areas and are absent in only four counties which have neither hospitals nor physicians – Rich, Piute, Wayne, and Daggett. Other data show that pharmacists are "even more dispersed into smaller communities within counties than are dentists and physicians," says the report, and then adds:

> ...Comparison of the number of pharmacies in the different counties and districts is difficult because data on size of pharmacies are not easily available. Thus it must be remembered that many pharmacies in the Wasatch Front are large operations, each employing many full-time pharmacists and open up to 24 hours a day, seven days a week, while in rural areas a pharmacy may be a one-man, part-time operation.

Pharmacists licensed by the state of Utah in 1972, according to *Utah Health Profile* (Utah State, 1973), were as follows:

County and Type of Area	*Number of Licensed Pharmacists*
Rural:	
Beaver	3
Daggett	0
Duchesne	5
Emery	2
Garfield	3
Kane	1
Millard	5
Morgan	2
Piute	0
Rich	0
San Juan	2
Sanpete	10

Summit	3
Wayne	0
Predominantly rural:	
Carbon	7
Sevier	10
Uintah	6
Predominantly urban:	
Box Elder	23
Cache	23
Davis	72
Grand	5
Iron	11
Juab	2
Salt Lake	350
Tooele	8
Utah	78
Wasatch	6
Washington	8
Weber	87
TOTAL	734

Distribution of dentists is a problem shared by all states in the Intermountain West. As seen in Table 7–9, Utah dentists in 1972 were distributed about the same as pharmacists, with heavy concentrations along the Wasatch Front counties and none in the four most rural counties. Table 7–10 gives a parallel picture of the distribution of dentists in Idaho, where there are but seventeen dentists in all of Idaho's fourteen rural counties — less than the total number of dentists in six individual counties which are predominantly urban. And Table 7–11 shows that, altogether, Montana's 32 rural counties have 46 dentists, the same number which can be found in Cascade County, which is only 13.3 percent rural. Montana's rural counties face this situtation in other areas of health care personnel (Montana State, 1974):

> While the three most populous counties [Yellowstone, Cascade, and Missoula]... account for less than one-third of Montana's total population, 49 percent of Montana's physicians are located in them, 42 percent of Montana's dentists, 41 percent of Montana's RNs, and 50 percent of the state's sanitarians. Furthermore, there are six counties in Montana with a total population of 9,765 which have no physicians. There are 13 counties with a total population of 30,067 which have no dentists.

Table 7-9

Distribution of Dentists in Utah[a]
(1972)

County and Type of Area	Dentists in Active Practice	Rate per Thousand Population
Rural:		
Beaver	2	0.49
Daggett	0	
Duchesne	2	0.21
Emery	1	0.19
Garfield	1	0.32
Kane	1	0.37
Millard	1	0.13
Morgan	2	0.46
Piute	0	
Rich	0	
San Juan	4	0.37
Sanpete	1	0.08
Summit	2	0.33
Wayne	0	
Predominantly rural:		
Carbon	4	0.24
Sevier	1	0.09
Uintah	3	0.20
Predominantly urban:		
Box Elder	17	0.57
Cache	18	0.40
Davis	33	0.31
Grand	2	0.32
Iron	8	0.62
Juab	2	0.44
Salt Lake	218	0.45
Tooele	6	0.32
Utah	61	0.41
Wasatch	4	0.62
Washington	8	0.50
Weber	65	0.49
TOTAL[b]	504	0.45

[a]Dentists listed in the yellow pages, including those in specialty practice.
[b]Includes 36 whose county of practice is unknown.

Source: Utah Center for Health Statistics, Division of Health, **Utah Health Profile** (Salt Lake City, December 1973).

Table 7-10

Distribution of Idaho's Dentists

(1971)

County and Type of Area	Dentists in Active Practice	Rate per Thousand Population
Rural:		
Adams	2	0.69
Blaine	2	0.35
Boise	0	
Butte	1	0.34
Camas	0	
Clark	0	
Custer	2	0.69
Jefferson	2	0.17
Lewis	1	0.25
Lincoln	2	0.66
Oneida	1	0.34
Owyhee	1	0.15
Teton	1	0.43
Valley	2	0.55
Predominantly rural:		
Bear Lake	3	0.51
Benewah	3	0.48
Bingham	8	0.27
Bonner	8	0.51
Boundary	2	0.31
Caribou	3	0.46
Cassia	6	0.35
Clearwater	3	0.27
Franklin	4	0.54
Fremont	2	0.23
Gem	2	0.21
Gooding	3	0.34
Idaho	7	0.54
Jerome	3	0.29
Kootenai	17	0.48
Minidoka	6	0.38
Payette	3	0.24
Shoshone	8	0.40

Table 7-10 (continued)

County and Type of Area	Dentists in Active Practice	Rate per Thousand Population
Predominantly urban:		
Ada	84	0.74
Bannock	34	0.65
Bonneville	39	0.76
Canyon	32	0.52
Elmore	4	0.22
Latah	9	0.36
Lemhi	3	0.54
Madison	5	0.37
Nez Perce	19	0.62
Power	3	0.62
Twin Falls	21	0.50
Washington	2	0.26

Source: Bureau of Health Resoures, Division of Manpower Intelligence, U.S. Department of Health, Education, and Welfare, **Area Resource File** (Rockville, Maryland, April 1974).

Table 7-11

Distribution of Montana Dentists

County and Type of Area	Dentists in Active Practice	Rate per Thousand Population
Rural:		
Blaine	2	0.29
Broadwater	1	0.40
Carbon	3	0.42
Carter	0	
Chouteau	2	0.30
Daniels	1	0.32
Garfield	0	
Golden Valley	0	
Granite	1	0.37
Jefferson	1	0.18

Table 7-11 (continued)

County and Type of Area	Dentists in Active Practice	Rate per Thousand Population
Judith Basin	0	
Lake	6	0.41
Liberty	0	
Madison	1	0.20
McCone	1	0.34
Meagher	1	0.47
Mineral	1	0.34
Musselshell	1	0.27
Petroleum	0	
Phillips	2	0.37
Powder River	0	
Prairie	0	
Ravalli	10	0.69
Rosebud	1	0.18
Sanders	2	0.28
Sheridan	3	0.52
Stillwater	2	0.43
Sweet Grass	1	0.33
Teton	2	0.32
Treasure	0	
Wheatland	1	0.40
Wibaux	0	
Predominantly rural:		
Big Horn	2	0.20
Flathead	28	0.71
Glacier	5	0.46
Lincoln	6	0.33
Pondera	3	0.45
Richland	3	0.30
Roosevelt	2	0.19
Nalley	6	0.52
Predominantly urban:		
Beaverhead	5	0.61
Cascade	46	0.56
Custer	5	0.41

Table 7-11 (continued)

County and Type of Area	Dentists in Active Practice	Rate per Thousand Population
Dawson	5	0.44
Deer Lodge	3	0.19
Fallon	1	0.25
Fergus	7	0.55
Gallatin	12	0.36
Hill	9	0.51
Lewis and Clark	19	0.57
Missoula	41	0.70
Park	7	0.63
Powell	3	0.45
Silver Bow	34	0.80
Tooele	2	0.33
Yellowstone	53	0.60

Source: Bureau of Health Resources, Division of Manpower Intelligence, U.S. Department of Health, Education, and Welfare, **Area Resource File** (Rockville, Maryland, April 1974).

Table 7–11 shows that there were ten counties without dentists in Montana in 1971. The quoted material above is taken from a 1974 source, thus it is shown that the lack of dental manpower in Montana has recently become more acute.

Throughout Nevada, the percentage of unfilled positions in 1972 for all professional and technical medical categories was 3.33 percent (Nevada State, May 2, 1974). For the two most populous counties, Clark and Washoe, unfilled positions are 3.38 and 3.16 percent respectively. For the rest of the state, which is almost entirely rural, if not by definition then by practicality, it is 3.97 percent.

Registered Nurses. Throughout the Intermountain Area the total number of registered nurses is minimal. A low count in physicians and hospitals brings a concomitant low count in registered and licensed practical nurses, as well as nurse's aides.

Wyoming's seven completely rural counties, Big Horn, Crook, Lincoln, Niobrara, Platte, Sublette, and Teton, had 32, eight, seventeen, twelve, seven, and 28 registered nurses respectively in

Table 7-12

Distribution of Registered Nurses in Wyoming (1972)

County and Type of Area	Number of Registered Nurses	Rate per Thousand Population
Rural:		
Big Horn	32	3.17
Crook	8	1.78
Lincoln	17	1.98
Niobrara	10	3.45
Platte	12	1.88
Sublette	7	1.89
Teton	28	5.83
Predominantly rural:		
Converse	22	3.73
Goshen	30	2.78
Weston	NA	
Predominantly urban:		
Albany	100	3.79
Campbell	24	1.86
Carbon	49	3.68
Fremont	88	3.11
Hot Springs	26	5.31
Johnson	19	3.39
Laramie	336	5.97
Natrona	273	5.33
Park	66	3.69
Sheridan	136	7.64
Sweetwater	79	4.34
Uinta	25	3.57
Washakie	28	3.76

NA = not available.

Source: Bureau of Health Resources, Division of Manpower Intelligence, U.S. Department of Health, Education, and Welfare, **Area Resource File** (Rockville, Maryland, April 1974).

1972 (State of Wyoming, 1974). Its five most urbanized counties – Sweetwater, Albany, Laramie, Natrona, and Washakie – had 79, 100, 336, 273, and 28 respectively. Two years later, all of the rural counties, except Teton and Niobrara, had many more people per nurse than the state ratio of 241:1, while all five of the more urban counties had more nurses to the population ratio than is recommended. Wyoming's registered nurses for 1972 are shown in Table 7–12.

On the surface, it would seem that Colorado ranks among the highest of all states in the Union in "almost all health manpower fields," according to a 1971 survey (Mueller, 1971):

> ...However, if one goes below the state level and looks at individual regions and areas within the state, a different situation exists. While certain areas in Colorado are well supplied with manpower, facilities, and services, others are not. In general, the rural areas which experience critical shortages of fundamental medical care services, i.e., physicians, dentists, and hospital services, lack most basic protective and preventive public health services as well.

Colorado's count of registered nurses by county for 1972 is as follows (U.S. Department of Health, Education, and Welfare, April 1974):

County and Type of Area	*Number of Registered Nurses*
Rural:	
Archuleta	0
Baca	17
Cheyenne	10
Clear Creek	3
Conejos	8
Costilla	5
Crowley	1
Custer	3
Dolores	0
Douglas	9
Eagle	15
Elbert	5
Gilpin	0
Grand	9
Hinsdale	0
Jackson	2

Kiowa	11
Lincoln	14
Mineral	1
Ouray	2
Park	8
Phillips	20
Pitkin	48
Rio Blanco	27
Routt	26
Saguache	6
San Juan	1
San Miguel	2
Sedgwick	13
Summit	5
Teller	8
Washington	9
Yuma	21
Predominantly rural:	
Bent	40
Chaffee	29
Delta	30
Garfield	69
Kit Carson	25
Mesa	282
Montezuma	42
Montrose	48
Rio Grande	38
Weld	384
Predominantly urban:	
Adams	549
Alamosa	46
Arapahoe	530
Boulder	593
Denver	5,108
El Paso	933
Fremont	69
Gunnison	16
Huerfano	16
Jefferson	673
Lake	29
La Plata	104
Larimer	361
Las Animas	35
Logan	84
Moffat	27
Morgan	52

Otero	74
Prowers	30
Púeblo	529

In Idaho and Nevada, registered nurses are also scarce. The following statistics for these states (U.S. Department of Health, Education, and Welfare, April 1974) shows the number of nurses in each county in 1972. Idaho's RNs per county range from 572 in Ada County to zero in Camas and Clark counties:

County and Type of Area	*Number of Registered Nurses*
Rural:	
Adams	10
Blaine	39
Boise	5
Butte	12
Camas	0
Clark	0
Custer	3
Jefferson	23
Lewis	12
Lincoln	8
Oneida	7
Owyhee	8
Teton	9
Valley	15
Predominantly rural:	
Bear Lake	11
Benewah	13
Bingham	77
Bonner	39
Boundary	13
Caribou	16
Cassia	30
Clearwater	30
Franklin	15
Fremont	32
Gem	25
Gooding	25
Idaho	30
Jerome	32
Kootenar	124
Minidoka	29
Payette	12
Shoshone	50

Predominantly urban:	
Ada	572
Bannock	230
Bonneville	216
Canyon	235
Elmore	43
Latah	96
Lemhi	10
Madison	29
Nez Perce	129
Power	15
Twin Falls	134
Washington	8

Nevada's number of registered nurses in 1972 ranged from one in Esmeralda County to 715 in Clark County. The *Area Resource File* gives the other county numbers as follows:

County and Type of Area	*Number of Registered Nurses*
Rural:	
Douglas	10
Esmeralda	1
Eureka	5
Lander	7
Lincoln	8
Lyon	17
Nye	11
Pershing	9
Storey	2
Predominantly rural:	
Churchill	25
Mineral	22
White Pine	16
Predominantly urban:	
Clark	715
Elko	42
Humboldt	14
Ormsby	32
Washoe	592

In Montana, three counties could not boast of a registered nurse in 1972 (U.S. Department of Health, Education, and Welfare, 1973): Golden Valley, Petroleum, and Treasure, all rural counties. The highest ratio of RNs to population was in Deer

Table 7-13

Distribution of Registered Nurses in Montana (1972)

County and Type of Area	Number of Registered Nurses	Rate per Thousand Population
Rural:		
Blaine	20	2.99
Broadwater	11	4.40
Carbon	13	1.86
Carter	7	3.68
Chouteau	20	3.08
Daniels	8	2.58
Garfield	5	2.73
Golden Valley	0	
Granite	13	4.81
Jefferson	11	2.08
Judith Basin	2	0.74
Lake	55	3.82
Liberty	10	4.35
Madison	23	4.60
McCone	9	3.10
Meagher	6	2.86
Mineral	11	3.79
Musselshell	9	2.43
Petroleum	0	
Phillips	11	2.04
Powder River	2	0.71
Prairie	10	5.88
Ravalli	42	2.94
Rosebud	18	3.00
Sanders	24	3.38
Sheridan	27	4.74
Stillwater	18	3.91
Sweet Grass	8	2.67
Teton	20	3.28
Treasure	0	
Wheatland	9	3.60
Wibaux	1	0.67

Table 7-13 (continued)

County and Type of Area	Number of Registered Nurses	Rate per Thousand Population
Predominantly rural:		
Big Horn	31	3.10
Flathead	125	3.17
Glacier	38	3.52
Lincoln	39	2.17
Pondera	34	5.15
Richland	33	3.37
Roosevelt	39	3.79
Valley	41	3.57
Predominantly urban:		
Beaverhead	17	2.10
Cascade	442	5.40
Custer	89	7.30
Dawson	36	3.19
Deer Lodge	117	7.55
Fallon	15	3.75
Fergus	58	4.60
Gallatin	164	5.05
Hill	89	5.11
Lewis and Clark	230	6.91
Missoula	296	5.08
Park	54	4.86
Powell	20	3.03
Silver Bow	247	5.87
Toole	18	3.05
Yellowstone	478	5.47

Source: Bureau of Health Resources, Division of Manpower Intelligence, U.S. Department of Health, Education, and Welfare, **Area Resource File** (Rockville, Maryland, April 1974).

Lodge County where there were 117 registered nurses per thousand population, or a rate of 7.55 nurses per thousand population (Table 7–13).

In Utah the number of registered nurses in 1972 was taken from statistical information cards sent out by the Utah Center for

Health Statistics. The following data reflect only those RNs who completed these cards. The total for the state was 2,900 RNs, divided as follows (Utah State, 1973):

County and Type of Area	*Number of Registered Nurses*
Rural:	
Beaver	12
Daggett	0
Duchesne	9
Emery	2
Garfield	5
Kane	5
Millard	14
Morgan	0
Piute	1
Rich	1
San Juan	18
Sanpete	14
Summit	3
Wayne	2
Predominantly rural:	
Carbon	51
Sevier	14
Uintah	15
Predominantly urban:	
Box Elder	45
Cache	100
Davis	103
Grand	11
Iron	25
Juab	8
Salt Lake	1,550
Tooele	28
Utah	310
Wasatch	14
Washington	13
Weber	522

Distance to Medical Care and Hospitals

Because there are fewer doctors in rural areas than in urban and suburban areas, it seems reasonable to conclude that rural residents must travel farther than city people for medical care.

However, in a report by the U.S. Department of Agriculture (1970), one statement stands out:

> ... Simple physical distance from available care is not a major impediment for most rural people. Hospital facilities of 25 beds or more are within a 25-mile distance of all but 8 percent of the rural population (compared with 2 percent of the total U.S. population).

But Erickson (1972), of the Mountain States Regional Medical Program, found that these national averages did not hold true for the Intermountain Region. In Wyoming, Montana, Nevada, and Idaho, only 17 percent of the population is within ten miles of a hospital, and 50 percent is at least 25 miles away. Says Erickson:

> While approximately 15 percent of the respondents for the entire region claimed they had to travel too far for medical care, almost half of all consumers whose households are in communities of 1,000 or less face this problem. These people normally travel out of state for medical care at a rate three times greater than do residents of communities with populations of 25,000 or more.

Travel in connection with illness is a financial drain; and in the case of hospitalization, this is true for both the patient and those who wish to visit him or her. In Colorado, according to Mueller (1971):

> The location of health resources and the time required for people to get there are important variables affecting health care, especially for rural Colorado. [Time is a much more relevant variable than distance in judging availability of health care. For example, to travel two miles through Metro Denver may take longer than to travel fifteen miles in rural eastern Colorado.] One-half of the state's population needs less than 15 minutes, 31.8 percent needs between 15 and 30 minutes, 10.7 percent needs one-half to one hour, and 3.9 percent needs over one hour to reach their physician's office. Compared to the other sources of health care, the distribution of physicians seems to be the best, and more time is required to reach the other health sources. For example, 13.5 percent of the state's population needs between one-half hour and one hour to reach a hospital, and 5.5 percent needs over one hour.

Over 48 percent of the households did not know how long it takes to reach a public health nurse. (Brackets are a footnote in the original.)

The predominantly rural areas of western Colorado are especially vulnerable to this problem. More than half of the residents of Dolores, San Juan, Montezuma, La Plata, and Archuleta counties must drive more than half an hour to reach their physicians, and over 26 percent need more than an hour to reach theirs. In addition, more than 30 percent must drive over an hour to get to the nearest hospital.

The Utah situation is no better. In the four "most rural" counties of the state, Daggett, Piute, Rich, and Wayne, a 26-mile drive is the least distance the residents must go to reach medical facilities (Table 7–14), according to *Utah Health Facts* (1972). While recognizing the fact that few people live in these rural areas, it also recognizes that "the few people who do, must travel great distances to the nearest physician; the nearest physician may even be in a neighboring state."

Sometimes the problem of distance can be looked at from a different point of view, as is the case with many of the rural people themselves, says Paul Westover,[7] health planner for southwestern Utah's Five-County Association of Governments. In Enterprise, Utah, for example, getting health care is a severe problem. Even when an emergency arises, people often must wait two to three hours. "If you were to ask them if they need a resident physician, they would say 'Yes, for emergency care.' But distance is not critical to them. The people have established their own patterns of health care, and many do not seek out care unless it is absolutely necessary. I know of people who will drive to St. George just to go bowling, and that's a hundred-mile round trip. Many do shopping in St. George and will have their health care needs taken care of then."

The rural people with whom Westover has worked are "just not used to seeking out health care," and this can disappoint a group who comes into an area wanting to remedy the lack of manpower or facilities. A lifetime of experience has taught many Intermountain rural residents to cope with the problem of distance to medical help, but there are also many who wish they didn't have

[7]Telephone interview, June 18, 1975.

Table 7-14

Distance Traveled by Citizens of Four Utah Counties to the Nearest Medical Facilities (1971)

County and Town or Community	Population	Nearest Facilities[a]	Miles
Daggett:			
Bridgeport	(b)	(c)	(b)
Dutch John	(b)	Vernal	43[d]
Green Lake	(b)	Vernal	40[e]
Manila	226	Vernal	69
		Green River (Wyoming)	45[e]
Piute:			
Angle	(b)	Panguitch	51
		Richfield	52
Circleville	443	Panguitch	27
		Richfield	53
Greenwich	25	Richfield	39
		Panguitch	64
Kingston	114	Panguitch	34
		Richfield	46
Marysvale	289	Richfield	32
		Panguitch	48
Rich:			
Garden City	134	Logan	40
		Montpelier (Idaho)	29
Laketown	208	Logan	53
Pickleville	106	Logan	43
		Montpelier (Idaho)	32
Randolph	500	Logan	73
		Ogden	86[d]
		Evanston (Wyoming)	32
		Kemmerer (Wyoming)	42

[a]All in Utah, except as shown in parentheses.

[b]Not given.

[c]Only back roads are available.

[d]Roads involved are reported by the Utah State Department of Highways as not plowed after each snowfall, and are thus less dependable in winter.

[e]Approximately.

Table 7-14 (continued)

County and Town or Community	Population	Nearest Facilities[a]	Miles
Sage Creek Junction	11	Logan	65
		Kemmerer (Wyoming)	34
		Evanston (Wyoming)	40
Woodruff	173	Ogden	76[d]
		Evanston (Wyoming)	22
		Kemmerer (Wyoming)	52
Wayne:			
Bicknell	264	Richfield	54
Caineville	(b)	Green River	78
		Richfield	98
Fremont	150	Richfield	47
		Panguitch	100
Grover	(b)	Richfield	70[e]
Hanksville	90	Green River	58
		Richfield	118
Loa	324	Richfield	47
		Panguitch	100
Lyman	170	Richfield	49
Teasdale	160	Richfield	64[e]
Torrey	84	Richfield	62
		Green River	114

Source: Utah Center for Health Statistics, Division of Health, **Utah Health Facts** (Salt Lake City, 1972).

to travel so far or take so much time to get to their doctor or to a hospital.

Problems in Pinedale, Wyoming. The town of Pinedale (population 948) is one of the Intermountain Region's small communities with the distance problem. Located in the only Wyoming county (Sublette) that has no in-patient care whatsoever, Pinedale is eighty miles from the hospital in Kemmerer, a hundred miles from Jackson, and a little over a hundred miles from Rock Springs. However, Pinedale has a clinic, a log cabin and former dance hall that was equipped in the 1940s with funds raised by open gambling.

"You won't find a more rural clinic anywhere else." says Pinedale's only doctor, Tom Johnston.[8]

Lillian Allen was born and grew up in this tiny hamlet not too far from the Grand Tetons. Her family has long been active in trying to get better medical care for the townspeople. Her brother-in-law Carroll Noble was the erstwhile owner of the log cabin which he donated to the town for the clinic. Ms. Allen has a clear memory of attempts to get Pinedale a hospital, including two bond levies, both of which were defeated.[9]

"There was rivalry between the two main towns in our county – Pinedale and Big Piney," she recalls. "Some thought Pinedale was the place for a hospital and others did not. Then there were people who maybe didn't like the doctor we had at the time, so they thought that if we didn't have a hospital he would leave. It was something I couldn't understand because there was so much need. We wanted a hospital with a nursing home attached, a place for small cases and emergencies, like it is in Jackson, so we wouldn't have to go out of the county. My mother spent seven and a half months in the hospital in Jackson and three months in Rock Springs. We just couldn't handle her ourselves because she was a large woman."

But there are always other points of view, such as Robert Smith's,[10] executive secretary of the Wyoming State Medical Society. "If you ask me, it would be a mistake to put a hospital in Sublette County... even though I know there are people there who really want one. Their population is such that they can't support a hospital. They have two good doctors – one in Pinedale and one in Big Piney. Both are GPs and do a good job, but a hospital there? No. A twenty-bed hospital in an area like Sublette would really create a problem. Have you ever tried to get good staff and equipment for a twenty-bed hospital? Sublette County is a perfect example of where a reliable form of transportation is needed to get [the people] to the health care center. And you can underline 'reliable' three times."

Rural Hospitals. Many other western towns share this dual problem of long distance to the nearest hospital and yet not enough people to adequately support one of their own. According to Health

[8]Telephone interview, March 5, 1975.

[9]Telephone interview, March 6, 1975.

[10]Telephone interview, March 11, 1975.

Systems Research Institute in Salt Lake City, Challis, Idaho, in Custer County has 784 residents, all of whom must travel at least 56 miles to the nearest hospital which is in Salmon. The four hundred citizens of Dubois, Idaho, must go 56 miles to Rexburg to get to a hospital. The 747 people living in Silverton, Colorado, have a thirty-bed hospital, but it is in such poor condition that it cannot be used. Therefore Silverton residents drive fifty miles over two mountain passes to Durango for any medical care because they have neither doctor nor hospital.

Oddly, many rural areas do have enough hospital beds. According to the U.S. Department of Agriculture (1973):

> Of the 7,123 hospitals in the United States in 1970, community hospitals constituted by far the largest number — 5,859 or 82 percent. The total number of hospitals was greater in rural than in urban areas. The number of beds per 100,000 population was also much larger in rural areas. Rural areas had 977.3 beds per 100,000 population, compared with 719.2 in urban areas.

In Nevada, for example, there is such an excess of hospital beds that strong indications point to a statewide occupancy ratio below 50 percent in the coming years. Say the Cooperative Health Planning officials (Nevada State, 1974):

> Excessive empty acute beds are the rule in most areas [of Nevada]. As of January 1, 1973, 2,500 acute beds were licensed by the Bureau of Health Facilities; an additional 273 beds were under construction at Washoe Medical Center. There were over 800 excess acute beds in the state at that time.

A primary reason that rural areas have a large number of hospitals is the 1946 Hospital Survey and Construction Act (Hill-Buton, discussed earlier). "Sparsely populated low-income rural and semirural counties have relatively more hospitals than do urban high-income counties, but the rural hospitals tend to be smaller and less adequately staffed" (U.S. Department of Agriculture, 1970).

The Committee on Government Operations (U.S. Congress, 1971) reports that the adequacy of hospital care can't "be measured by the number of beds relative to the population to be served or by the number of hospitals." People in rural areas are "hampered by small hospitals which are not as well staffed with technical personnel and are poorly equipped." In many of these hospitals, medical staff organization policies, necessary to meet the quality standards of the Joint Commission on Accreditation of Hospitals, are lacking. Many have no outpatient departments, "a significant deficiency in the provision of adequate services.... While there may be an emergency room, such a service does not meet the need for regular medical care for the rural poor," says the report, and continues with:

> Hospitals that serve large populations can usually afford to acquire needed equipment. If this is not possible, they can often share equipment with other hospitals in the same general area. Such an arrangement tends to lessen the financial burden to metropolitan hospitals. In nonmetropolitan areas, however, hospitals are so far apart that a hospital is forced to obtain its own equipment, or go without. This heavy capital investment coupled with low occupancy rates, which range from 70 percent to 80 percent, combine to keep rural hospitals in debt. A minimum occupancy of 90 percent is necessary to keep hospitals from losing money.... The problem of accessibility and acceptability directly relate to the low occupancy rate at which nonmetropolitan hospitals operate. Many are very difficult to reach, thereby discouraging people from making visits except in times of severe duress. In addition, many facilities in nonmetropolitan areas are so antiquated that potential patients will not use them. Since 1963, health care facilities which do not adhere to the provisions of Title VI if the Civil Rights Act, providing equal access for all persons regardless of race, religion, or place of national origin, are not eligible for new money from the Hill-Burton program. Nonadherence to Title VI also prohibits health care facilities from participating in the Medicare and Medicaid programs. Lack of federal construction money leads to quick obsolescence; lack of Medicare and Medicaid money raises hospital fees as well as limits access for most of the rural poor, who are not covered by private insurance and cannot afford hospital expenses.

Other Intermountain Hospital Statistics. Nevada's entirely rural counties have no hospital immediately available and the other five rural counties have one hospital each (Table 7–15). The bed ratio per hundred thousand population is fairly high in those rural counties that do have hospitals. However, the quantity of services

Table 7-15

Proportion of Beds per Thousand Population in Nevada Hospitals (1970)

County and Type of Area	Number of Hospitals		Beds per Thousand Population
	General	Other	
Rural:			
Douglas	0	0	
Esmeralda	0	0	
Eureka	0	0	
Lander	1	0	6.15
Lincoln	1	0	10.77
Lyon	1	0	5.12
Nye	1	0	4.55
Pershing	1	0	18.08
Storey	0	0	
Predominantly rural:			
Churchill	1	0	4.04
Mineral	2	0	10.14
White Pine	1	0	8.61
Predominantly urban:			
Clark	7	1	3.22
Elko	2	0	6.40
Humboldt	1	0	7.46
Ormsby	1	0	4.94
Washoe	3	1	7.41

Source: Bureau of Health Resources, Division of Manpower Intelligence, U.S. Department of Health, Education, and Welfare, **Area Resource File** (Rockville, Maryland, April 1974).

offered is not so high. According to the September 1970 data in the *Area Resource File* (U.S. Department of Health, Education, and Welfare, April 1974), Lander County had a blood bank, extended care, a hospital auxiliary, and an organized outpatient department. Lincoln County had intensive care and intensive cardiac units, a nursery for premature babies, a blood bank, a part-time registered pharmacist, and physican and inhalation therapists. Lyon County offered intensive cardiac care, a recovery room, extended care, and a hospital auxiliary. Nye County had a blood bank, extended care, and an organized outpatient department. Pershing County had intensive cardiac care, a recovery room, extended care, and a hospital auxiliary.

None of these counties had X-ray therapy, radium therapy, occupational therapy, dialysis (outpatient or otherwise), psychiatric care, social workers, rehabilitation (outpatient or otherwise) – all available in urban Clark and Washoe counties.

A Nevada certified public accountant told the Federal Price Commission of the problems of six of his client county hospitals in sparsely populated areas (Nevada State, July 1974). All provided acute and nursing home care to patients in small communities, had 75 or fewer beds, and were the only hospitals in their particular town.

> ...They are all experiencing trends toward decreasing occupancy and, with the exception of one, all are marginal operations from a financial standpoint. All experienced net operating losses in 1972, and most have suffered losses for several years, after considering building and equipment depreciation. The counties involved are unable to provide additional financial support to those hospitals because they themselves are in poor financial condition and are uniformly assessing the maximum lawful property tax.

In addition, several counties in Nevada have hospital beds that do not conform to state or federal standards. In 1972, Lyon County was licensed for 24 general acute beds, none of which met state or federal standards. Pershing County was licensed in 1972 for 22 general acute care beds and 25 licensed skilled nursing beds, none of which met standards. Both of these counties are 100 percent rural according to the *Area Resource File.*

Also, in the predominantly but not 100 percent rural Nevada areas, twelve of Churchill County's 42 general acute care beds did not conform with federal standards, and ten of Mineral County's 25 general beds did not conform. In the most urban counties, 298 of Clark's 1,555 acute care beds did not meet standards, and 214 of Washoe County's 916 general acute care beds did not conform. While the more urban counties had some beds that did not meet with all standards, they all had some, and usually many, beds that did meet them.

One of the reasons that rural hospitals are often inadequate, says Hollis K. LeFever,[11] a rural practitioner in Lewistown, Montana, and past president of the Montana Medical Association, is that a large percentage of rural people lack confidence in their local facilities and in their medical personnel. Many rural residents go once a year or even every two years to a medical center in a large city. Bypassing local facilities means that the facilities cannot be developed to provide good medical care.

"The very best doctor going into a rural practice faces this problem, and I don't think it is justified," said Dr. LeFever. "The solution rests in part with the centers that see our people occasionally. If they discredit the local facilities, they are discrediting them in the eyes of the local residents. For example, a patient with diabetes goes to a large center where his disease is well controlled; he is on a strict diet, and his activity is limited. So the doctor reduces his insulin and when the patient comes back home, he doesn't watch his diet and he exercises more vigorously than he should, and I have to increase his insulin. The same with hypertension. These people get back in their home surroundings, away from a low-salt diet and back to family tensions. The same with GI tract patients.

"When the medical center doctor alters the prescription, he should explain to the patient, 'I am seeing you under unusual circumstances. Be sure that you continue to check with your home doctor.' This would result in two things; first, it would be an insurance that the prescription would continue to be good and, second, it would reflect confidence in the local doctors. But they [the medical center doctors] don't, and I have to get up at one a.m. and go down to the emergency room. A change in attitude on the part of the big medical center's personnel would really help. A lot of people haven't even seen the rural areas and they discredit the facilities."

In Tables 7–16, 7–17, and 7–18, the proportion of hospital beds per thousand population for Colorado, Idaho, Montana, and Utah, and the number of hospitals and hospital beds for Wyoming are shown. Table 7–16 gives the category "other" (hospitals), while Tables 7–17 and 7–18 show only "number of hospital beds" because the tables were adapted from three different sources. Nevertheless, one can see the paucity of hospital beds in the rural, pre-

---

[11]Telephone interview, April 3, 1975.

dominantly rural, and many times in the predominantly urban areas of these Intermountain states.

Table 7-16

Proportion of Beds per Thousand Population in Colorado, Idaho, and Montana Hospitals (1970)

State, County, and Type of Area	Number of Hospitals		General Hospital Beds per Thousand Population
	General	Other	
Colorado:			
Rural			
Archuleta	0	0	
Baca	1	0	4.46
Cheyenne	1	0	12.92
Clear Creek	0	0	
Conejos	1	0	4.10
Costilla	0	0	
Crowley	0	0	
Custer	0	0	
Dolores	0	0	
Douglas	0	0	
Eagle	0	0	
Elbert	0	0	
Gilpin	0	0	
Grand	1	0	4.88
Hinsdale	0	0	
Jackson	0	0	
Kiowa	1	0	9.00
Lincoln	1	0	8.33
Mineral	0	0	
Ouray	0	0	
Park	1	0	3.64
Phillips	2	0	1.00
Pitkin	1	0	4.92
Rio Blanco	1	0	1.00
Routt	1	0	3.03
Saguache	0	0	
San Juan	0	0	
San Miguel	0	0	

Table 7-16 (continued)

State, County, and Type of Area	Number of Hospitals		General Hospital Beds per Thousand Population
	General	Other	
Colorado (continued)			
Sedgwick	1	0	7.65
Summit	0	0	
Teller	1	0	3.64
Washington	1	0	7.82
Yuma	2	0	5.29
Predominantly rural			
Bent	1	1	6.56
Chaffee	1	0	8.32
Delta	1	0	1.84
Garfield	1	0	4.46
Kit Carson	1	0	5.87
Mesa	6	0	8.97
Montezuma	1	0	6.36
Montrose	1	0	3.04
Rio Grande	2	0	8.56
Weld	2	0	4.30
Predominantly urban			
Adams	2	1	1.69
Alamosa	1	0	8.42
Arapahoe	1	1	2.83
Boulder	3	1	2.53
Denver	12	11	8.73
El Paso	6	2	5.26
Fremont	3	0	9.36
Gunnison	1	0	2.67
Huerfano	1	0	5.85
Jefferson	1	1	1.37
Lake	1	0	4.51
La Plata	2	0	8.13
Larimer	2	0	1.97
Las Animas	0	0	
Logan	1	0	7.23
Moffat	1	0	4.62
Morgan	2	0	4.45
Otero	2	0	5.34
Prowers	1	0	4.02
Pueblo	2	1	6.07

Table 7-16 (continued)

State, County, and Type of Area	Number of Hospitals		General Hospital Beds per Thousand Population
	General	Other	
Idaho:			
Rural			
Adams	1	0	6.90
Blaine	2	0	7.54
Boise	0	0	
Butte	1	0	7.59
Camas	0	0	
Clark	0	0	
Custer	0	0	
Jefferson	0	0	
Lewis	0	0	
Lincoln	0	0	
Oneida	1	0	3.79
Owyhee	0	0	
Teton	1	0	5.65
Valley	2	0	9.44
Predominantly rural			
Bear Lake	1	0	6.03
Benewah	1	0	5.97
Bingham	1	1	1.71
Bonner	1	0	2.58
Boundary	1	0	8.13
Caribou	1	0	10.77
Cassia	1	0	3.35
Clearwater	1	1	2.41
Franklin	1	0	2.19
Fremont	2	0	5.17
Gem	1	0	5.27
Gooding	1	0	3.14
Idaho	2	0	4.57
Jerome	1	0	7.84
Kootenai	1	0	3.60
Minidoka	1	0	3.80
Payette	0	0	
Shoshone	2	0	5.18
Predominantly urban			
Ada	3	1	4.79
Bannock	3	1	5.49

Table 7-16 (continued)

State, County, and Type of Area	Number of Hospitals		General Hospital Beds per Thousand Population
	General	Other	
Idaho (continued)			
Bonneville	2	0	6.93
Canyon	2	1	4.36
Elmore	2	0	3.37
Latah	1	1	2.41
Lemhi	1	0	7.09
Madison	1	0	2.24
Nez Perce	1	0	3.40
Power	1	0	9.38
Twin Falls	2	0	3.84
Washington	1	0	3.95
Montana:			
Rural			
Blaine	1	0	3.28
Broadwater	1	0	9.20
Carbon	1	0	7.29
Carter	1	0	19.47
Chouteau	1	0	6.00
Daniels	1	0	12.58
Garfield	1	0	11.67
Golden Valley	0	0	
Granite	1	0	3.70
Jefferson	0	0	
Judith Basin	0	0	
Lake	3	0	8.54
Liberty	1	0	4.78
Madison	2	0	4.60
McCone	1	0	6.90
Meagher	0	1	
Mineral	1	0	7.24
Musselshell	1	0	8.92
Petroleum	0	0	
Phillips	1	0	5.74
Powder River	0	0	
Prairie	1	0	11.76
Ravalli	1	0	2.24
Rosebud	1	0	3.33
Sanders	1	0	2.25

Table 7-16 (continued)

State, County, and Type of Area	Number of Hospitals		General Hospital Beds per Thousand Population
	General	Other	
Montana (continued)			
Sheridan	1	0	5.61
Stillwater	1	0	5.87
Sweetgrass	1	0	5.67
Teton	1	0	3.61
Treasure	0	0	
Wheatland	1	0	0.31
Wibaux	0	0	
Predominantly rural			
Big Horn	2	0	6.20
Flathead	2	0	2.69
Glacier	2	0	8.33
Lincoln	1	0	1.89
Pondera	1	0	7.12
Richland	1	0	5.51
Roosevelt	3	0	9.13
Valley	1	0	6.70
Predominantly urban			
Beaverhead	1	0	2.22
Cascade	3	1	7.72
Custer	2	0	19.02
Dawson	1	0	4.07
Deer Lodge	1	1	6.77
Fallon	1	0	6.25
Fergus	1	0	6.98
Gallatin	1	0	3.20
Hill	1	0	8.91
Lewis and Clark	3	1	11.56
Missoula	3	0	6.19
Park	1	0	5.23
Powell	1	0	5.30
Silver Bow	2	0	8.12
Toole	1	0	11.02
Yellowstone	1	0	4.62

Source: Bureau ofHealth Resources, Division of Manpower Intelligence, U.S. Department of Health, Education, and Welfare, **Area Resource File** (Rockville, Maryland, April 1974).

Table 7-17

Proportion of Beds per Thousand Population in Utah Hospitals (1971)

County and Type of Area	Beds in General Hospitals	
	Number	Per Thousand Population
Rural:		
Beaver	26	6.8
Daggett	0	
Duchesne	32	4.1
Emery	0	
Garfield	14	4.4
Kane	22	8.8
Millard	40	5.6
Morgan	0	
Piute	0	
Rich	0	
San Juan	56	5.5
Sanpete	34	3.0
Summit	13	2.2
Wayne	0	
Predominantly rural:		
Carbon	70	3.2
Sevier	22	2.1
Uintah	34	2.6
Predominantly urban:		
Box Elder	37	1.3
Cache	118	2.7
Davis	74	0.4
Grand	38	6.0
Iron	49	3.8
Juab	31	6.7
Salt Lake	1,686	3.6
Tooele	38	1.7
Utah	423	2.9
Wasatch	25	4.0
Washington	41	2.8
Weber	523	4.1

Source: Center for Health Statistics, Division of Health, **Utah Health Profile** (Salt Lake City, 1973).

Table 7-18

Number of Hospitals and Hospital Beds in Wyoming (1974)

County and Type of Area	Number of General Hospitals	Number of General Hospital Beds
Rural:		
Big Horn	2	60
Crook	1	16
Lincoln	2	35
Niobrara	1	24
Platte	1	43
Sublette	0	
Teton	1	38
Predominantly rural:		
Converse	1	32
Goshen	1	44
Weston	1	42
Predominantly urban:		
Albany	1	93
Campbell	1	31
Carbon	1	85
Fremont	2	111
Hot Springs	1	50
Johnson	1	26
Laramie	2	316
Natrona	1	298
Park	2	89
Sheridan	1	89
Sweetwater	1	97
Uinta	1	22
Washakie	1	36
TOTAL	27	1,678

Source: Wyoming State Office of Comprehensive Health Planning, Division of Health and Medical Services, **Wyoming Health Profile, 1974** (Cheyenne, 1974).

Emergency Medical Services

Better emergency medical services are another item needed in many rural areas where long distances between towns and cities prohibit the immediate care needed in life and death situations.

Training people within the community would be of help, says Dr. Harris Knudson,[12] a radiologist associated with Las Vegas' Southern Nevada Memorial Hospital and chairman of the Commission of Medical Practice of the Nevada State Medical Society. Dr. Knudson feels that many of these efforts have been "messed up" by politics, however, and that the medical community should be involved in planning emergency medical services, using the knowledge that it already has of the situation. A particular irritation to Knudson is that so much money is spent on studies, but few plans are actually put into action. "I think I've seen a quarter of a million dollars go down the drain within the last few years by studying things to death," he states.

Many of the specific problems facing the emergency medical services system in Nevada are summarized below (Nevada State, vol. I, 1973). Several points apply to the entire Intermountain Region.

(1) Vast distances, often made treacherous by mountainous terrain and foul weather
(2) One of America's highest violent death rates
(3) Less than one ambulance per thousand square miles
(4) A lack of coordination between the elements on the front line of emergency care; i.e., hospital emergency departments, air and ground ambulances, law enforcement agencies
(5) Major shortages and maldistribution of health manpower
(6) Nonexistent communications between ambulances and emergency rooms
(7) Lack of adequate training and other "software" programs
(8) Lack of legal statement of responsibilities in providing emergency health services
(9) Lack of regulatory authority concerning ambulance equipment
(10) A lack of funds for proper training and equipment and for communications improvement
(11) Only seven emergency facilities service 72 percent of the state's area, with each one serving an average of ten thousand square miles

---

[12]Telephone interview, March 16, 1975.

Coverage of large areas by a small number of ambulance services, in (3) above, is an especially acute one in Nevada and elsewhere in the Intermountain Area. In 1972 there were 56 ambulance services in Nevada, according to the state's emergency medical plan (Nevada State, vol. II, 1973). Thirteen were either military, industrial, or associated with two U.S. Public Health Service hospitals. The remaining 43 ambulance services covered 109,889 square miles and served the general public. Ambulance services in states that border Nevada do take patients to Nevada hospitals but rarely pick up patients in Nevada. An exception is an ambulance service located on the north shore of Lake Tahoe.

Nevada had 27 licensed acute hospitals in 1972. One did not accept emergency patients, four were federal hospitals, and one was the state mental hospital. This left 21 hospitals open as general service facilities providing emergency services to the public at large. In addition, a major emergency department – with holding beds – served the area around the Nevada test site.

Only 108 ambulances operated in the state in 1972, less than one for each thousand square miles. The vast distances between hospitals can best be understood by the following:

- Tonopah is 208 miles from Las Vegas.
- Caliente and Las Vegas are 150 miles apart.
- Ely is 187 miles from Elko.
- Fallon is 257 miles from Ely.
- Seven rural hospitals serve an area of more than seventy thousand square miles.

Thus it can be seen that, in Nevada, immediate medical services are often unavailable to the sufferer.

Each of the other Intermountain states has problems similar to Nevada's, although the ratio of population to square miles differs. Wyoming's clusters of settlements, towns, and cities leave great distances between outlying settlements and available hospitals. Idaho, Montana, and Colorado, even though their population rates are higher, still have rural communities that are far from emergency medical help.

Utah is one of the Intermountain states that has made early progress in emergency medical services. Salt Lake City's Intermountain Regional Medical Program became involved before the Emergency Medical Care Act of 1973. According to Lionel Drage,[13]

[13]Personal interview, February 19, 1975.

director of emergency medical services for Utah's program, the Act guided Utah into better emergency medical services before "everyone really got into the emergency medical care routine."

In 1972, says Drage, Utah's Intermountain Regional Medical Program received a $475,000 grant enabling it to place primary ambulances in almost every community and to equip them with four-channel, high-band radios. This allowed a twofold benefit: (1) every hospital in the state is now able to communicate with the ambulances, and (2) the ambulances are able to communicate with the hospitals while in transit. "Suppose the ambulance is transporting a man and he starts to hemorrhage," says Drage. "They can get in touch with the closest hospital and tell them the problem and ask them to have a doctor there when they arrive."

Each hospital in Utah's nine emergency districts was also provided with in-band repeaters by which they can communicate with other hospitals in their districts. "These are to be used for physician consultation, to get supplies such as blood from nearby hospitals, and for disaster purposes," says Drage.

As a final part of the emergency plan, the program's Emergency Medical Services Division made three contracts. The first was with the Utah Ambulance Association. Its purpose was to study all of the rural ambulances to determine what equipment they were lacking and to set up priorities as to needs. The ambulances were then provided with essential equipment that was lacking. The second contract was with the Utah State Division of Health and was to train ambulance drivers as emergency medical technicians by giving them the standard 81-hour emergency course. The third was an agreement with the Utah Hospital Association, by which all of the emergency rooms in rural hospitals were studied and, again, priorities set up and needed equipment furnished by the program.

Drage says that the 1973 Emergency Medical Services law will eventually bring emergency care systems similar to Utah's to all of the states. Millions of dollars in funds are being given out during this three-year law. Excellence in all programs was required at first, but now that time is running out, and as the government wants all the states to start some sort of emergency plan, less comprehensive programs are being allowed.

Current emergency medical services efforts are now being concentrated on the training of more ambulance drivers, upgrading and replacing obsolete ambulances, and retraining rural nurses. The program has put three rural nurse-training programs into action, training the nurses partially at the University Medical Center in Salt Lake City and partially in the rural areas.

Recently the Intermountain Regional Medical Program received a $340,000 grant from the Robert Wood Johnson Foundation, to assist rural areas in designing and implementing a single emergency phone system. This will coordinate and become a part of the state emergency medical services system.

"The program is also working on providing fixed wing ambulance service to rural Intermountain areas," says Drage. Currently, there is one such program available through Intermountain Aviation in Salt Lake City, but problems have been many. For one thing, few doctors know about its availability, thereby making utilization low and the price high; for another, there is a lack of equipment. Still another problem is the need to develop the manpower to operate the service. The program has trained forty physicians and nurses in air ambulance transportation of the sick and injured, but the program needs better coordination to improve the rate of utilization. "Right now, the highest rate of utilization is the elective transfer," says Drage, giving an example of that as being "when someone in Cedar City wants to transfer Aunt Sadie to a rest home in Salt Lake.

"There are problems with air transportation that you don't encounter in an ambulance on the ground. You take off from St. George, which is a certain elevation [3,800 feet], and then go up twelve thousand feet over the mountain and that causes problems that the technician doesn't know how to handle. He's competent, but he just hasn't faced this situation before." Drage explained that the high altitude can cause such problems as spurting I.V.s or that "a person with a catheter in him is going to get mighty uncomfortable when he's up that high."

The airplane service has been around for fifteen years, and is much better than it once was, despite problems encountered. Although it is currently based only in Salt Lake City, Drage hopes that qualified airplanes throughout the Intermountain Region can be used. "Shared services is what will make it successful," he prophesies.

Selected References

Cooper, James; *et al.* "The Decision for Rural Practice." *Journal of Medical Education* (December 1972), vol. 47.

DuVal, Merlin K., M.D. "A Program for Rural Health Development." *Journal of the American Medical Association* (July 10, 1972), vol. 221, no. 2.

Erickson, Donald L. "Consumer Health Education: A Rural Renaissance." *Rocky Mountain Medical Journal* (December 1972).

Graves, Constance L., M.D.; *et al.* "Anesthesia in the Intermountain Region." *Rocky Mountain Medical Journal* (February 1968).

Montana State Division of Comprehensive Health Planning. *Montana State Plan for Health.* Helena: Department of Health and Environmental Science. August 1974.

Mueller, Heinz F., M.A. *Colorado Health Consumer Survey — A Regional Analysis: Colorado-Wyoming Regional Medical Program.* Denver: Colorado Office of Comprehensive Health Planning and Colorado-Wyoming Regional Medical Program. May 1971.

Nevada State Allied Health Manpower Inventory and Planning Estimates for 1975 and 1980. *Comprehensive Health Planning.* Summary extract. May 2, 1974.

——— Cooperative Health Planning in Cooperation with the Office of Highway Safety. *Nevada Emergency Medical Services Plan.* Volumes I and II. March 1973.

———. *Nevada State Plan for Acute and Long-Term Care Health Facilities.* July 1974.

President's National Advisory Commission on Rural Poverty. "People Left Behind." Washington, D.C.: President's National Advisory Commission on Rural Poverty. 1967.

U.S. Congress, Senate, Committee on Government Operation. *The Economic and Social Condition of Rural America in the 1970s: Inpact of Department of HEW Programs on Nonmetropolitan Areas, 1970.* 92d Cong., 1st Sess. May 1971.

U.S. Department of Agriculture. *Rurality, Poverty, and Health.* Agricultural Economic Report No. 172. Washington, D.C.: U.S. Department of Agriculture. February 1970.

______________, Rural Development Service. *Health Services in Rural America.* Agriculture Information Bulletin No. 362. Washington, D.C.: U.S. Government Printing Office. July 1973.

U.S. Department of Commerce, Bureau of the Census. *Number of Inhabitants, U.S. Summary.* Washington, D.C.: U.S. Government Printing Office. 1970.

______________. *Statistical Abstract of the United States, 1973.* Washington, D.C.: U.S. Government Printing Office. 1973.

U.S. Department of Health, Education, and Welfare, Health Resources Administration. *Area Resource File.* Rockville, Maryland: Division of Manpower Intelligence, Bureau of Health Resources. April 1974.

______________, Public Health Service. *Health Characteristics by Geographic Region....* Rockville, Maryland: National Health Center. January 1974.

Utah State Department of Social Services, Division of Health. *Utah Health Facts.* Salt Lake City: Center for Health Statistics. May 1972.

______________. *Utah Health Profile.* Salt Lake City: Center for Health Statistics. December 1973.

Wyoming State Division of Health and Medical Service. *Wyoming Health Profile, 1974.* Cheyenne: Office of Comprehensive Health Planning. 1974.

8

Rural Life – More Hazardous Than Healthy

The statistics on rural versus urban health manpower and facilities in chapter 7 indicate that rural residents in the Intermountain Region – indeed, throughout most of the United States–have less access to medical care than urban dwellers. One might ask: Do rural residents *need* more medical facilities and more doctors than they already have? Perhaps this chapter can help answer this question.

In this modern era, it appears to be a common belief that the "wholesome" country life is also a healthy one as people dream of a house in the country, leave the city to go backpacking in the forests and mountains, or try to get "back to the farm" by at least starting a vegetable garden. However, the odds are against their finding *healthful* living in rural areas because of a dearth of medical facilities and practitioners and the fact that, in rural areas, there is not a sufficient economic base to establish such facilities within easy distance of many rural residents.

Rural health problems and rural income intertwine in an ever-expanding circle that engulfs the families who live on farms. It is because rural incomes are generally lower and medical services usually poorer and less accessible than they are in the city that the incidence of chronic illness – which limits work activity and

Table 8-1

Percentage Distribution of Men 27 to 34 Years of Age Who Did or Did Not Qualify for Military Service, by Place of Origin[a]

(1964)

Place of Origin	Examined	Qualified: Served	Qualified: Did Not Serve	Rejected	Not Examined
Large cities of a hundred thousand or more	90%	71%	7%	12%	10%
Suburbs of large cities	87	70	5	13	13
Cities of 25,000 to 99,999	87	67	4	12	13
Town or small city of less than 25,000	86	68	4	14	14
Rural areas:					
Nonfarm	84	58	3	23	16
Farm	82	55	6	21	18

[a]Residence during childhood and adolescence before age fifteen; may not total 100 percent because of rounding.

Source: Rural Development Service, U.S. Department of Agriculture, "Health Services in Rural America," Agricultural Information Bulletin No. 362 (Washington, D.C.: U.S. Department of Agriculture, July 19, 1973).

thus reduces income — increases both in rural families and in low-income families, indicating a need for additional services (U.S. Department of Agriculture, 1970). Farmers in general experience a high rate of this type of chronic illness.

One of the many examples of poor rural health is shown in Table 8–1, wherein it can be seen that of those who were examined for military service in 1964 — men 27 to 34 years of age — and whose place of residence was determined according to where they lived during childhood and adolescence, military rejection was least for those in cities, and almost twice as high for those in the rural areas (U.S. Department of Agriculture, 1973).

It is difficult to document that people living in rural Intermountain Area counties have more cases of chronic disease than those who live in urban counties. A county with a small total population is more likely to have a smaller number of people afflicted with any one disease than would a country with a large population; this lower incidence makes rates less stable for comparison purposes. One additional death will hardly affect a rate based on two hundred deaths, but it will double a rate based on only one death. According to the *Montana State Plan for Health* (Montana State, 1974):

> ... [It] is possible for a county with a small population to "luck out" and have low rates for all of the variables selected as health status indicators. For deaths from a specific cause (for example, lung cancer) a county with a small population will either have a rate of zero if there were no deaths from that cause ... or a relatively high rate if there was even one death from this cause during the period.

Thus it is difficult to prove conclusively that individual rural counties have high rates of chronic ailments. However, it can be documented that older people do have high rates, as seen in Figure 8.1. It can also be shown that rural counties have a large percentage of elderly population.

Diseases, Chronic and Acute

As farms and ranches have become larger, their need for workers has been for fewer but more highly skilled men. Therefore young adults migrate from the rural areas to look for available work, or perhaps to attend college, or for other opportunities they feel urban life has to offer. This removes people from the rural areas who are in their most productive years, people who work and pay taxes and whose buying power might help attract health care personnel. Left are the elderly, who have a large percentage of the chronic ailments, and also the very young, who suffer from a majority of the acute illnesses (discussed later).

Table 8–2 reveals that the Intermountain Region's rural area has a lower percentage of people over the age of 65 than does the rural United States as a whole (10.1 percent of all U.S. rural residents are 65 or over, while the Intermountain Region's rural residents over age 65 make up 8.8 percent of the population). Also,

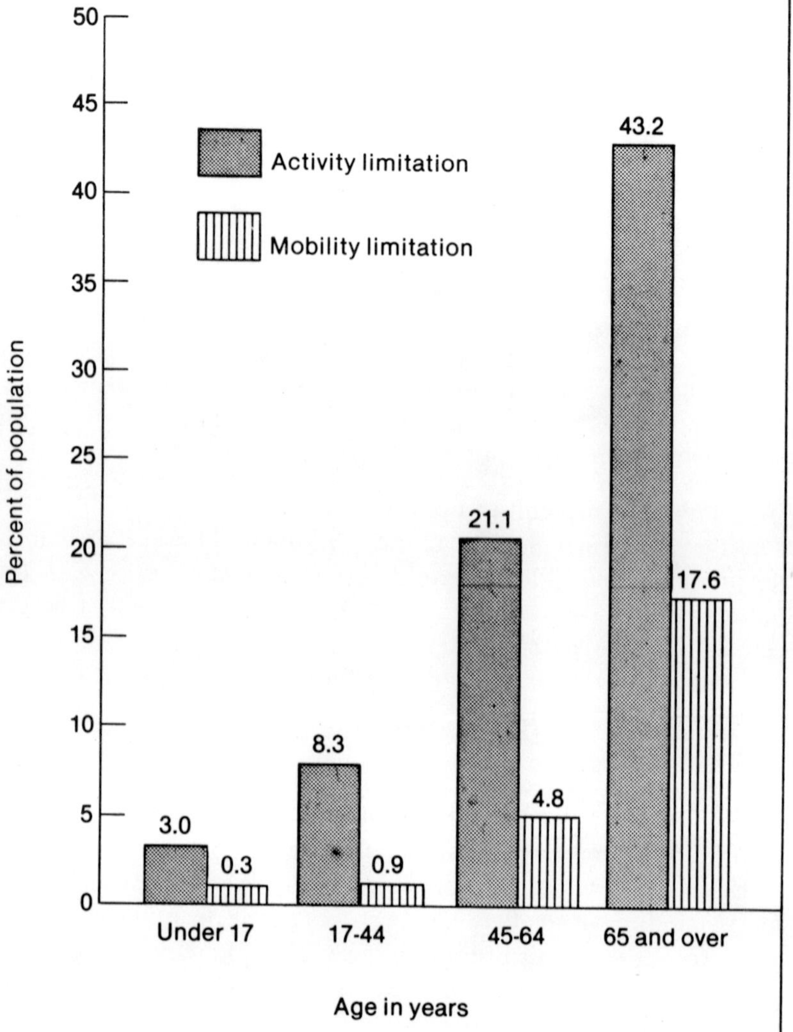

Source: National Center for Health Statistics, Rockville, Maryland.

Figure 8.1. Percentage of Population with Limitation of Activity or Mobility due to Chronic Condition, by Age, 1972

Table 8-2

Age Distribution of Urban-Rural Population in the Intermountain Region and the United States (1970)

State or Area	Urban				Rural			
		Percentage				Percentage		
	Median Age	Over 21	Under 18	Over 65	Median Age	Over 21	Under 18	Over 65
Colorado	25.9	59.2%	34.3%	8.4%	27.5	58.0%	37.7%	8.8%
Idaho	26.1	58.4	34.9	10.2	26.9	56.6	39.3	8.7
Montana	26.3	58.6	34.9	9.9	28.0	60.0	38.3	9.9
Nevada	27.7	60.9	34.6	6.2	28.5	60.2	35.9	6.9
Utah	23.1	54.2	39.2	7.2	23.0	52.3	43.1	8.0
Wyoming	26.9	59.1	34.7	9.4	27.7	58.0	38.2	8.6
All states in Intermountain Region		58.2	35.5	8.3		57.1	38.8	8.8
United States	28.1	61.0	33.3	9.8	27.9	58.7	36.8	10.1

Source: Bureau of the Census, U.S. Department of Commerce, **Census of the Population, 1970,** vol. I, parts 1, 7, 14, 28, 30, 46, and 52 (Washington, D.C.: U.S. Government Printing Office, 1970); Bureau of the Census, U.S. Department of Commerce, **Summary, Colorado, Idaho, Montana, Nevada, Utah, and Wyoming** (Washington, D.C.: U.S. Government Printing Office, 1973).

when the six states are averaged, there are only 0.5 fewer percentage points of urban residents over age 65 than rural. But Utah, Nevada, and Colorado all have a slightly higher percentage of people over 65 living in the rural areas. Montana's percentage is the same for urban and rural (9.9 percent), and the other two states have fewer rural people over age 65.

Surprisingly, even though the percentage points are not far apart, the median ages for the rural areas are higher in all of the states except Utah, which has a young population in both the rural and urban regions. And when counties are taken individually, it can be seen that many of the rural ones have a high percentage of elderly people. While Table 8–3 points out that Wyoming as a whole has 9 percent of its population over the age of 65 (which is less than the national percentage of 9.9), nine of its counties are over both the state and national level, and only three are urban. Two of the urban counties, in fact the county with the highest percentage of population over 65 and the county with the third highest, are classified urban but have 36.7 and 38.7 percent rural population.

Wyoming has a median age for the state of 27.2, which is lower than the national median of 28.3, but sixteen counties were over the state average (five were rural) and eleven were over both the national and state average. Considering that Wyoming has 23 counties, this leaves seven counties to pull the average down to 27.2; thus some counties must have a young median age. The two youngest counties are Albany and Campbell (percentage of rural population is 12.8 and 44.1 respectively), followed by Fremont with 46.6 percent rural population. Another county with a rather young population is Laramie, which is the home of the state capital of Cheyenne and also a state university where students are counted in the census. Laramie county, with 19.5 percent of its population being rural, has a median age of 26.7.

Discussing age distribution in Utah's counties, the *Utah Health Profile* (1973) says:

> Nine counties in the state have greater percentages of people over 65 than they do in the 15–19 cohort. These same counties also have less than the state average percentage in the one to 14 age cohort. Such distribution could be caused by outmigration of younger people and by inmigration of 65 and over persons. As all nine of these counties are predominantly

Table 8-3

Wyoming's Median Age and Percentage of Population over Age 65 (1974)

County and Type of Area	Over Age 65	Median Age
Rural:		
Big Horn	12.9%	31.5
Crook	8.6	27.4
Lincoln	9.2	26.7
Niobrara	15.5	37.6
Platte	13.8	33.3
Sublette	6.3	26.9
Teton	5.9	27.4
Predominantly rural:		
Converse	12.8	30.2
Gosher	13.2	31.8
Weston	9.4	27.4
Predominantly urban:		
Albany	6.1	23.3
Campbell	4.8	23.3
Carbon	9.6	29.7
Fremont	6.8	25.5
Hot Springs	16.5	36.3
Johnson	12.9	31.6
Laramie	8.4	26.7
Natrona	7.5	26.3
Park	8.7	27.7
Sheridan	15.9	36.8
Sweetwater	9.6	29.0
Uinta	10.3	29.3
Washakie	8.3	27.7
All of Wyoming	9.0	27.2
United States	9.9	28.3

Source: Division of Health and Medical Service, **Wyoming Health Profile, 1974** (Cheyenne: Office of Comprehensive Health Planning, 1974).

rural, with inherently few employment opportunities, the forced move to employment opportunities causes outmigration and the population distributions exhibited by nine counties.

These nine counties are Beaver, Emery, Juab, Kane, Millard, Piute, Sanpete, Sevier, and Wayne, which according to the *Area*

Resource File are all 100 percent rural except for Juab (33.3 percent) and Sevier (54.4 percent).

Another age factor that can indicate a high percentage of health problems is a large percentage of children – the ones who usually suffer most from acute diseases, as is shown in Figure 8.2. The Intermountain population in rural areas has 3 percent more persons under the age of eighteen than does the nation's rural areas. All six states have a higher percentage of people under age eighteen in the rural population than in the urban, as was shown

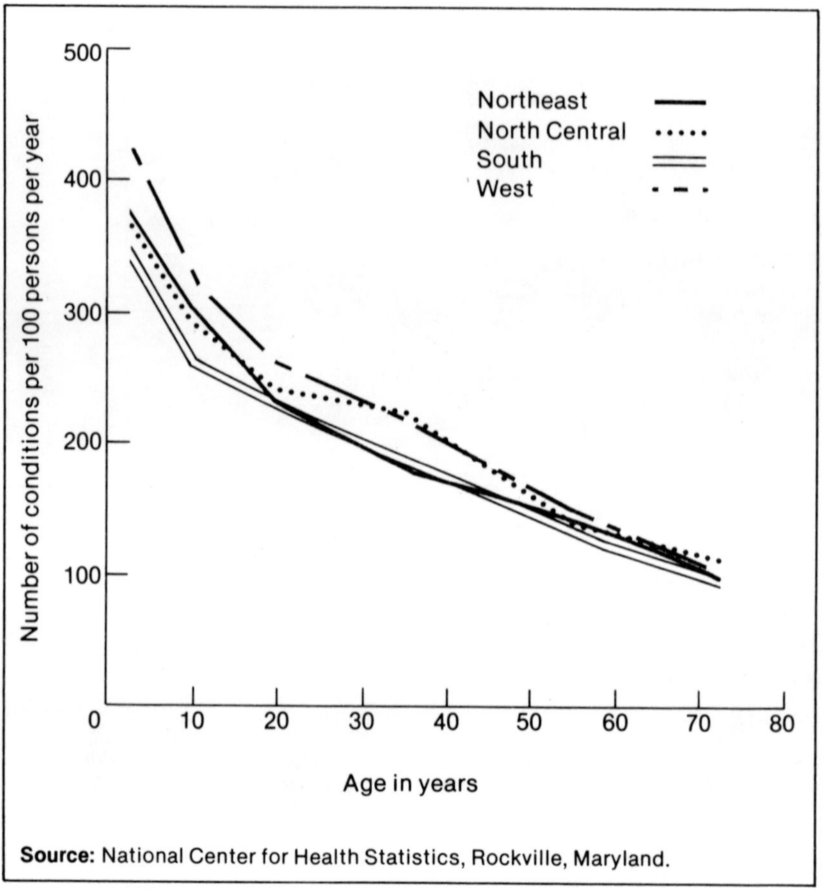

Figure 8.2. Incidence of Acute Conditions per Hundred Persons per Year by Geographic Region and Age, July 1971 to June 1972

in Table 8–2. Utah in particular has a young population, with a median age of 23 in the rural areas and 23.1 in the urban. Of Utah's rural population, 43.1 percent are under age eighteen, while 39.2 percent of its urban residents are under eighteen.

Infant Mortality

One fairly good barometer of health is infant mortality rates, and these are available for most of the Intermountain states. According to Ford (1964):

> Infants are particularly prone to disease arising from poor environmental health conditions as is evident in their higher rates of death from contagious diseases, digestive disorders arising from unsanitary food and water supply, and malnutrition. Consequently the infant mortality rate [number of deaths of infants under one year of age per thousand live births] has long served as one of the more sensitive indexes of health conditions. The tremendous improvements in the health status of the United States population is clearly evident in the decline in infant mortality since 1915. In that year the infant mortality rate for the death registration states was 99.9, or one infant death for every ten births; in 1961 the rate was 25.3, or one death for approximately every forty births.

The 1973 infant mortality rate was 17.6.

Nevada, which is very much a rural state except for the populated areas near Reno and Las Vegas, has not only a high birth rate, indicating need for services, according to *Preventive Health Services* (Nevada State, 1974), but also a higher infant mortality rate and a higher maternal mortality rate than the U.S. average. Approximately 2.5 percent of all Nevada pregnancies in 1973 resulted in fetal or infant death, and 8.7 percent of all Nevada children born that year were subject to impairments due to low birth weight. If one combines these two figures, it appears that one out of every ten pregnancies resulted in death or a high probability of impairment. However, this statement may be misleading in that many of the infant and fetal deaths might have been included in the low birth rate group.

In Montana, infant death rates in 1968–72 for those counties with large populations rated in the low quartile, except for Silver Bow (Montana State, 1973). The majority of infant deaths in the medium high and high quartiles are in the rural and predominantly rural counties, as seen below; but it must be remembered that the small rural populations contribute to small rates and thus are not good comparisons. Therefore it would probably be best to compare 1972 rates in Colorado, readily available by districts, making the population and the rates more stable. The following are the figures for Montana's five-year infant mortality rate by place of residence for 1968 to 1972.

County and Type of Area	*Mortality Rate per Thousand Live Births*
Rural:	
Blaine	25.9
Broadwater	18.2
Carbon	26.9
Carter	6.7
Chouteau	27.2
Daniels	20.9
Garfield	7.4
Golden Valley	13.3
Granite	22.3
Jefferson	28.6
Judith Basin	35.3
Lake	24.1
Liberty	11.7
Madison	23.0
McCone	17.3
Meagher	38.5
Mineral	35.7
Musselshell	18.7
Petroleum	0.0
Phillips	22.8
Powder River	26.2
Prairie	14.2
Ravalli	22.9
Rosebud	18.6
Sanders	18.1
Sheridan	13.8
Stillwater	10.6
Sweet Grass	17.5
Teton	14.2
Treasure	21.3
Wheatland	15.2
Wibaux	0.0

County and Type of Area	*Mortality Rate per Thousand Live Births*
Predominantly rural:	
Big Horn	24.5
Flathead	21.3
Glacier	21.0
Lincoln	23.0
Pondera	24.9
Richland	13.9
Roosevelt	39.2
Valley	24.0
Predominantly urban:	
Beaverhead	24.5
Cascade	16.9
Custer	19.4
Dawson	13.9
Deer Lodge	27.6
Fallin	30.9
Fergus	20.3
Gallatin	21.3
Hill	9.7
Lewis and Clark	21.4
Missoula	20.0
Park	21.0
Powell	27.1
Silver Bow	26.7
Toole	17.4
Yellowstone	17.5

In Colorado, of thirteen planning districts, eight of which are 50 percent or more rural, the four with the highest rate of infant mortality were rural, as seen in Table 8–4. However, the four with lowest rates of infant mortality were also rural, with the five more urban counties all in the middle. The state average mortality rate was 17.6; four of the rural and four of the urban districts were higher than this, although the difference was much greater for the rural ones.

In Utah in 1970, of the fourteen entirely rural counties, eight had infant mortality rates higher than the rate for the state as a whole, which was 15.0. Seven of these rural counties had the highest rate in the state (Table 8–5). If one discounts those counties with no infant deaths (five of the six with no death rates were in rural counties, probably because of small rates in sparsely populated

Table 8-4

Colorado's Infant and Neonatal Deaths
(1972)

Area	Infant Deaths		Neonatal Deaths	
	Number	Rate	Number	Rate
District:				
1[a]	13	13.7	11	11.6
2	58	18.2	43	13.5
3	361	17.7	262	12.4
4	103	18.5	73	13.1
5[a]	7	28.8	5	20.2
6[a]	12	13.5	5	5.6
7	37	16.8	29	13.1
8[a]	11	16.5	6	9.0
9[a]	16	24.2	11	16.6
10[a]	14	21.7	9	14.0
11[a]	16	28.0	12	21.0
12[a]	16	28.0	12	21.0
13[a]	11	18.1	8	13.2
All of Colorado	678	17.6	487	12.6

[a]Fifty percent or more rural.

Source: Colorado Planning and Management District, **Demographic Profile;** 1 to 13 prepared by Colorado Department of Health Records and Statistics Section, Statistics Unit, September 20, 1973.

areas), one sees that of the ten lowest rates, five were in urban areas, three were in counties predominantly rural (50 percent or more, but not 100 percent), and two were in rural counties.

Neonatal mortality (deaths of infants four weeks of age or younger) is also an excellent indicator of health conditions. Says Ford (1964):

> A high ratio of newborn to total infant deaths is generally considered an index of good health conditions on the assumption that many of the newborn deaths are unavoidable because of congenital defects, but a higher proportion of the deaths of older infants could be prevented by proper health and medical care.

Table 8-5

Utah's Infant and Neonatal Death Rates by County of Mothers' Residence

(1970)

County and Type of Area	Infant Mortality		Neonatal Mortality	
	Deaths	Rate	Deaths	Rate
Rural:				
Beaver	3	33.7	2	22.5
Daggett	0		0	
Duchesne	8	44.0	6	33.0
Emery	1	10.5	1	10.5
Garfield	3	49.1	0	
Kane	2	36.4	1	18.2
Millard	1	7.7	1	7.7
Morgan	3	32.2	3	32.2
Piute	0		0	
Rich	0		0	
San Juan	11	36.5	6	19.8
Sanpete	4	18.9	4	18.9
Summit	3	21.3	3	21.3
Wayne	0		0	
Predominantly rural:				
Carbon	3	11.1	1	3.2
Sevier	1	5.0	0	
Uintah	4	13.3	3	10.0
Predominantly urban:				
Box Elder	7	11.2	5	8.1
Cache	14	11.5	6	4.9
Davis	40	16.4	34	14.0
Grand	1	6.9	1	6.9
Iron	3	9.7	3	9.7
Juab	2	18.9	2	18,9
Salt Lake	170	14.9	129	11.3
Tooele	10	18.4	6	11.0
Utah	61	14.0	49	11.3
Wasatch	0		0	
Washington	11	29.9	7	19.0
Weber	39	12.6	28	9.1
All of Utah	405	15.0	301	11.2

Source: Utah State Division of Health, **Utah Health Profile** (Salt Lake City: Center for Health Statistics, July 1972).

Table 8-6

Montana's Infant and Neonatal Deaths and Rates (1973)

County, State, and Type of Area	Infant Deaths		Neonatal Deaths	
	Number	Rate	Number	Rate
Rural:				
Blaine	2	15.5	2	15.5
Broadwater	0		0	
Carbon	2	18.7	0	
Carter	0		0	
Chouteau	2	26.0	0	
Daniels	1	20.0	1	20.0
Garfield	1	33.3	1	33.3
Golden Valley	1	62.5	0	
Granite	0		0	
Jefferson	5	53.2	4	42.6
Judith Basin	0		0	
Lake	2	7.5	2	7.5
Liberty	1	34.5	1	34.5
Madison	0		0	
McCone	0		0	
Meagher	2	52.6	2	52.6
Mineral	1	14.1	1	14.1
Musselshell	1	30.3	1	15.2
Petroleum	0		0	
Phillips	2	25.6	2	25.6
Powder River	0		0	
Prairie	0		0	
Ravalli	5	23.3	3	14.0
Rosebud	6	37.5	4	25.0
Sanders	4	35.4	4	35.4
Sheridan	0		0	
Stillwater	0		0	
Sweet Grass	0		0	
Teton	0		0	
Treasure	0		0	
Wheatland	3	83.3	1	27.8
Wibaux	0		0	
Predominantly rural:				
Big Horn	6	27.1	2	9.0
Flathead	12	20.0	8	13.3
Glacier	6	25.0	3	12.5
Lincoln	3	9.3	3	9.3
Pondera	4	36.4	3	27.3

Table 8-6 (continued)

County, State, and Type of Area	Infant Deaths		Neonatal Deaths	
	Number	Rate	Number	Rate
Richland	2	11.1	1	5.6
Roosevelt	10	48.1	7	33.7
Valley	5	19.6	3	11.8
Predominantly urban:				
Beaverhead	1	9.4	1	9.4
Cascade	30	21.2	21	14.9
Custer	3	15.9	3	15.9
Dawson	2	12.0	2	12.0
Deer Lodge	2	9.2	2	9.2
Fallin	1	15.4	1	15.4
Fergus	3	20.5	3	20.5
Gallatin	12	24.6	11	22.5
Hill	3	10.4	1	3.5
Lewis and Clark	10	17.9	7	12.5
Missoula	14	14.2	8	8.1
Park	2	11.6	2	11.6
Powell	2	18.7	1	9.3
Silver Bow	18	27.9	14	21.7
Toole	0		0	
Yellowstone	29	19.8	19	13.0
All of Montana	222	19.5	155	13.6

Source: Montana State Department of Health and Environmental Science, **Annual Vital Statistics Report, 1973** (Helena: Bureau of Records and Statistics, 1973).

Tables 8–4 and 8–5 show differences among counties, but, again, one must look at Colorado's rates because of the information by districts and hence the higher rates of occurrence and more stability for comparison. In 1972, according to Table 8–4, of the predominantly rural counties, the difference of percentage points between infant deaths and neonatal deaths was roughly 2, 8, 8, 7, 8, 7, 4, and 7; while the six more urban districts had a span of 5, 5, 5, 3, and 5 points. Difference in percentage points can be seen in Table 8–6 for Montana and 8–5 for Utah.

Accidents

Accidents play a large role in health problems of Americans, both rural and urban. They are the fourth largest killer in both the United States and the Intermountain Region, preceded only by heart disease, cancer, and stroke. According to *Preventive Health Services* (Nevada State, 1974):

> The National Center for Health Statistics and the National Safety Council estimate that as a result of home injuries each year, 30,000 people are killed; 110,000 are permanently disabled, and 585,000 are hospitalized; and more than 20 million are injured seriously enough to require medical treatment or to be disabled for a day or more. Most of these casualties are associated with consumer products.

A high percentage of accidents occur to rural residents, especially those in the western states, as shown in the following figures (from the National Center for Health Statistics) for the United States and the West (number of persons per one hundred thousand injured each year):

Geographic Region	*Number Injured*
United States:	26.3
SMSA –	26.0
Central city	24.7
Outside central city	27.0
Large SMSA	27.3
Other SMSA	25.2
Outside SMSA –	27.0
Nonfarm	27.7
Farm	22.1
West:	32.8
SMSA –	31.8
Central City	30.5
Outside central city	31.4
Large SMSA:	32.7
Los Angeles	35.7
San Francisco	25.0
Other SMSA	29.5
Outside SMSA –	38.3
Nonfarm	38.5
Farm[1]	

[1]Because there is more than a 30 percent relative standard error, the number injured for the "farm" category does not meet standards of reliability or precision.

Excluded from the above statistics are all conditions involving neither restricted activity nor medical attention.

According to the *Wyoming Emergency Medical Services* (Wyoming State, 1971):

> The leading cause of death in our young people aged one to 37 is accidental injury. The price tag on accidental injury has been estimated at $18 billion yearly. One out of every four Americans suffers an accident every year. Traffic accidents account for 10 percent of the total.... In the past 60 years, more Americans have died from accidental injury than from combat wounds of all our wars. Accidental injury has been termed our foremost environmental health problem.

The very nature of rural occupations, particularly farming, makes rural residents prone to accidental injury. Farming is the third most dangerous occupation today. According to Powers (1958), until 1955 agriculture was annually responsible for more occupational deaths than any other major industry. Accidents occur during routine farm chores and include mishaps with small but potentitally hazardous implements — tools, scythes, axes, pitchforks, manure forks — and with high-powered, dangerous machinery such as tractors, mowing machines, power takeoffs, and corn pickers. Rural residents are also inclined to accidents due to falls, farm animals, and pesticides and other agricultural chemicals. Waller (1967) tells of one study which

> ...has shown that a substantial proportion of farmers, housewives, and students do not understand the terms most commonly used on the labels of agriculture and home products. This problem exists for the most part because of ignorance by the manufacturer or the distributor, rather than because of lack of concern.

Another factor in farm accidents is the lack of safety promotion in the agriculture business. According to Coe (1959), the history of safety in industry goes back to the early 1900s, but it was not until 1944 that agricultural safety began to receive adequate attention. During that year, the National Farm Safety Committee was set up in the National Safety Council and attention was focused on the farm accident problem.

In the largely agricultural Intermountain Region, the same theme holds true — farming is a hazardous business. In Idaho in

1973, the greatest number of the 48 occupational deaths were sixteen in agriculture, as seen below in data from the Idaho State Department of Health and Welfare, Bureau of Vital Statistics, for occupational accidental deaths.

Occupation	*Number of Deaths*
Agriculture	16
Mining, quarrying, oil and gas wells	–
Logging and lumber industry	11
Construction	4
Transportation	5
Other and unspecified industry	12
TOTAL	48

The third highest category, after "other and unspecified," were eleven deaths in the logging and lumbering industry – neither an urban pursuit.

In Wyoming in 1970, agricultural deaths ranked highest in the occupational category. The second highest was the combined category of mining, quarrying, oil and gas wells – with six deaths. Total number of Wyoming deaths occurring at work in 1970 was thirty. The figures below are from the Wyoming Division of Health and Medical Services, *Wyoming Vital Statistics, 1967–70*, for occupational accidental deaths, 1970.

Occupation	*Number of Deaths*
Agriculture	11
Mining, quarrying, oil and gas wells	6
Construction	4
Manufacturing and public utilities	2
Transportation	2
Trade	–
Service	2
Government	–
Other and unspecified	3
TOTAL	30

In Utah in 1973, agriculture was a comparatively safe business — that is, at least it was the fifth largest killer, rather than number one. According to the Utah Safety Council's report, *Utah Accident Facts, 1973*, accidental deaths for occupations were as follows:

Occupation	*Number of Deaths*
Agriculture	5
Mining, quarrying, oil and gas wells	6
Construction	10
Manufacturing and public utilities	9
Transportation	1
Service	7
Other and unspecified	3
TOTAL	41

Altogether, the Intermountain states look like an unsafe place to live. According to *Montana Vital Statistics* (Montana State, 1972):

> Montana has historically had a high death rate from accidents, and 1972 was particularly a bad year. The 635 deaths produced a death rate of 88.3 per 100,000 population, which was up from 1971 (85.8) and was the third highest rate in the last 20 years.

The death rate for the nation for that year, due to accidents, was 54.6. In Utah in 1970, 58.3 persons per hundred thousand lost their lives because of accidents, while the U.S. rate was 54.2 that year (Utah State, 1972). Idaho had a high rate in 1973 of 75.2, according to *Idaho Vital Statistics* (1973); and Colorado's was slightly lower than that year's national rate of 54.8, with a rate of 54.2 (Colorado State, 1973). Generally, the rate of deaths due to accidental causes is greater in the Intermountain Region than in the nation as a whole.

Traffic Fatalities and Injuries

Traffic accidents make up a large percentage of rural accidental deaths. According to *Rural Health News* (1975):

> While the majority of the nation's population is urban in residence, the majority of highway fatalities are rural in

occurrence. Rural roads and highways are the sites for about seven out of every ten traffic fatalities. The fatalities include both rural and urban residents who often die not because of the irreversible severity of their injuries, but because care is inadequate and not immediately available. More than 6,000 farm residents each year die as a result of farm, home, and highway accidents. The growth of recreation centers and tourism in rural areas makes the problem more acute.

Waller did abundant research on rural automobile accidents, using California as the site of many studies. One such study (Waller, 1967) showed that

> ...although half of the fatalities in both urban and rural areas were primarily from head injuries, in the majority of rural head injuries, brain tissue was not injured, whereas in most of the urban fatalities, there was brain injury. It is suspected that many of those injured in rural areas died simply because they choked to death from blood, mucous, etc., in the mouth and windpipe.

In 1969 Waller quoted another study, saying that

> ...for most types of injury resulting in death, those injured in rural areas more frequently died within the first hour. For example, of persons in urban crashes whose major cause of death was from chest injury, 59 percent died during the first hour, compared to 75 percent among those who died of similar injuries in rural crashes. Furthermore, of all persons injured in urban areas who died during the first hour, only 37 percent died at the site of the injury, whereas in the rural areas, 90 percent of those who died during the first hour were still at the crash site. It is highly relevant that the more rapid death of those injured in rural crashes *cannot* be explained by a greater inherent severity of such crashes, because in the fatal urban crashes 53 percent of the injuries believed to have caused death were determined to be probably nonsurvivable, whereas in the rural crashes, 38 percent of such injuries were probably nonsurivable.... In a study of rural ambulance services, we found that almost a quarter of patients carried were nonresidents. Another study shows that 32 percent of highway fatalities in rural counties were nonresidents, in comparison to 12 percent of fatalities in urban counties. Between the hours of midnight and 6 a.m., 42 percent of those fatally injured in rural areas were nonresidents.

Many of the more serious crashes, Waller found, are commonly associated with alcohol and occur when the traffic is lightest:

> . . . [Of] drivers and pedestrians who had alcohol in their blood at the time they were fatally injured, two thirds had crashed between the hours of 9 p.m. and 6 a.m. The use of alcohol among the fatally injured is similar in both urban and rural crashes. . . . It is relevant that such crashes, because they tend to occur when traffic is lightest, also more commonly involve only a single vehicle. Consequently, a longer time may elapse between injury and discovery. Single vehicle crashes are more common in areas with low population density because in such areas traffic, even at its worst, is not as heavy. This is one possible explanation for greater case-fatality ratio associated with rural crashes. Also extremely important is the fact that the most serious crashes tend to occur during hours when in all except very large cities, staffing is least adequate in hospitals, police departments, ambulance companies, and other emergency units.

A study in California comparing the injury-fatality rates of rural county residents with urban residents, found that residents of individual rural counties in some cases were ten times more likely to die of injury (Waller, 1969).

In fact, according to *Wyoming Emergency Medical Services* (Wyoming State, 1972) 70 percent of traffic fatalities occur in areas of less than 2,500 population and the death rate for injuries of similar severity is four times higher in rural than urban areas. Waller (1967) says, "in general, the less populated states appear to have higher fatality rates per 100,000 population."

Nevada, with a density of one person per square mile or less throughout most of the state, is a good example of this. From 1971 through 1973, approximately 49 percent of all accidental deaths in the United States were due to motor vehicle accidents, while in Nevada during that same time, the percentage was 60 (Nevada State, 1974).

Motor vehicle accidents far outled other types of accidental deaths in Utah in 1968–70, with 53.1 percent of all fatalities, and falls being a distant second at 13.8 percent. The highest traffic fatality rate in the state per ten thousand 1970 resident population was 54.7 in Juab County (33.3 percent rural) and the lowest, 5.3, in Davis county (13.7 percent rural). Salt Lake County was second lowest, with a rate of six per ten thousand. Both the highest and lowest percentage of fatal accidents were in rural counties, with Emery at 76 percent and Kane at 25 percent. Those counties are both entirely rural (Utah State, 1972).

Wyoming, according to the Governor's Office of Highway Safety, had 195 deaths in 1974 due to traffic accidents, and only 27 of them were in urban areas. In 1970, Wyoming lost 194 persons for the same reason, with 182 from rural places.

In Montana, which has a high rate of deaths due to accidents, 50.1 of the 88.3 rate per hundred thousand population in 1972 was for traffic fatalities (Montana State, 1972). In 1974, Montana had a total of 8,397 traffic accidents in rural areas and 258 deaths, while urban areas suffered 7,363 accidents and 41 deaths. There were 5,613 rural persons injured and 2,850 urbanites injured, with 1,698 incapacitating rural injuries and 541 incapacitating urban injuries (Montana State, 1974).

Mental Illness

There is another hazard in rural life, and while it is not as visible as an automobile accident, it has as much potential to maim rural residents as does a speeding car. This danger is mental illness.

In 1963, Congress recognized the growing problem of mental illness and passed the Community Mental Health Centers Act. This established and funded mental health centers throughout the country. All have at least five basic services: in-patient services, out-patient services, partial hospitalization (such as day or night care), emergency services 24 hours a day, and consultation and educational services. There are other clinics and hospitals that work toward mental health, but without these five basic requirements they are not federally funded community mental health centers.

According to the report by the U.S. Department of Health, Education, and Welfare (1971), of the 295 community mental health centers in 1971, 175 or 59.3 percent served urban areas, 87 or 29.5 percent served partially rural areas, and only 33 or 11.2 percent were for rural residents.

"I have a theory about rural mental illness," says Dorthea Dolan,[2] recently retired special assistant for rural mental health

[2]Telephone interview, March 25, 1975.

at the National Institute of Mental Health in Rockville, Maryland. "Mind you, it's just a theory, but then it's probably as good as any other theory.

"If the incidence of new mental illness cases is the same in rural as in urban communities, unless spontaneous remissions equal incidence, there must be a higher prevalence in rural areas, as you would get an accumulation of untreated mental illness in rural areas because they have a dearth of treatment centers.... There may be a greater tolerance to mental illness in rural areas; we don't know. But we do know that the resources in the rural areas do not compare with those in the urban areas, and I have no evidence that the rural people have less need."

Dolan compares it with treating tonsilitis: "While city and rural children probably both have tonsilitis at about the same rate, the urban children have more access to doctors and treatment and are more likely to have their tonsils taken out than the rural child. And you can't get tonsilitis without tonsils."

In other words, those who have treatment available to them use it more often and have a much better chance of recovery.

As reported by Kraenzel and Macdonald (1971), a study of eighteen rural Montana counties done from January 1, 1963, to July 1, 1965, revealed that the admission rate to the state hospital for these counties was less than that of two urban counties of similar size, but that were located nearer the hospital. "This was especially so when compared with the population nearest the hospital. Also, those admitted to the state hospital from the areas nearer the hospital were admitted more often than those from the more rural areas; that is, there were more readmissions." The researchers felt that there was "little doubt" but what many of the former patients in the rural areas would have sought more help had there been a local service or if the state hospital had been more accessible.

"Because most psychiatric patients have been shown treatable without hospitalization," believes Cohen (1972), "outpatient services constitute a key element in a community mental health program." Yet rural centers provide only about half as many cases of outpatient care annually as their non-rural counterparts (Jones, *et al.*, 1974).

Intermountain Community Health Centers. Utah's 84,916 square miles have six community mental health centers, one serving a rural population and one having special problems of caring for both urban and rural residents (Utah State, 1975). The Four Corners Community Mental Health Center, extremely rural, stretches its staff over 17,492 miles and 37,000 people in the eastern part of the state. There are two offices, one in Price and one farther south in Moab.

The Murray–Jordan–Tooele Community Mental Hygiene Center serves 130,000 people in the suburban sprawl of southern Salt Lake County and continues through Tooele County to the Nevada border. A small permanent clinic in Tooele has been established to help with the needs of the rural residents.

Sixteen of Utah's 22 counties, many of them rural, do not have community mental health centers, although half have been given the approval for centers but not yet the funds. These areas are covered by "mental health specialists," and until future centers come, these few specialists are "it" to many rural people.

For the most part, they work alone, spending about 75 percent of their time with adults, including follow-up for former state hospital patients. In some areas, their efforts are bolstered by traveling mental health teams of psychiatrists, psychologists, and nurses who visit their counties two days a month and work primarily in schools.

The specialists coordinate programs with other agencies, work in the schools, give direct services, answer midnight emergency calls, handle acute patients who must be sent to the state hospital and follow up on them when they return home. And with the variety of the job, they see a variety of problems.

One such problem is depression, perhaps common in rural areas. George Brinkerhoff is a mental health specialist who works in the central part of the state. He says that there is a unique kind of depression a farmer faces when his children do not want to farm and he has to give up land that has been in his family for generations. Only half facetiously he calls it the "I-don't-want-to-give-up-the-farm-to-somebody-from-California-syndrome."

The state of Idaho has been divided into seven regions, each having a community health center that offers the five basic services. Six are state-run and one is private, but all receive government funds. These main centers are in Coeur d'Alene, Lewiston, Nampa-Caldwell, Boise, Twin Falls, Pocatello, and Idaho Falls, and all have at least two to six satellite clinics that offer as many services as they can, says Joy Buersmeyer,[3] executive director of the Mental Health Association of Idaho. Only the Boise Clinic could be classified as an urban one, she added. "I think we have got them as strategically located as we can. People may have to drive a bit, but that's better than having to come up all the way to Boise. But there is still a stigma attached to mental illness and I think that is more of a deterrant from getting care than is the distance."

According to Dolly Emerson,[4] secretary with the Southwest Montana Mental Health Center, Montana has five community mental health centers in the state's larger communities of Butte, Great Falls, Miles City, Billings, and Missoula, with anywhere from four to six satellite clinics reaching out to the smaller and more rural towns.

"Colorado is doing well," says Dolan. "They have eleven centers in all. The sixteen counties in northwest Colorado are covered, and there are also centers in the San Louis Valley, Greeley, Jefferson, and Arapahoe counties."

Wyoming, she says, has a rural center in the northeast corner of the state with headquarters in Sheridan. There are also centers in Cheyenne and one in Fremont County. "By definition, that county [Fremont] is urban, but we serve the people," says Dolan, "and the people are rural."

Nevada is the only state in the nation, besides Connecticut, that does not have a National Institute of Mental Health center in its rural counties; but where Connecticut has only one rural county, the situation in Nevada is almost reversed. "There are two Nevada centers in the urban counties of Washoe and Clark where Reno and Las Vegas are, but the rural people in the remaining hundred thousand square miles are not served by a Community mental health center," said Dolan, adding that there are some state and local facilities, however.

At least one study (Jones, *et al.*, 1974) has found that the rural community health centers that do exist are of an "extraordinary nature." But there are problems, too. The shortage of centers is coupled with shortage of personnel, plus the fact that almost two-thirds of the staff at nonrural and partly rural centers are full-time, in contrast to approximately 40 percent in rural community mental health centers. "Over half of the staff in the latter category are

---

[3]Telephone interview, July 17, 1975.

[4]Telephone interview, July 18, 1975.

part-time, with a very small proportion of trainees and volunteers," says Jones.

The supply of personnel is also badly distributed, says Dolan. "You can find personnel on the East coast and in California, but there is not a fair share in the rural areas.

"I recently called some of the rural centers west of the Mississippi, and I found ninety vacancies for psychiatrists. These are all budgeted positions; there is money for them, but they are still vacant. And this is a minimum need because I didn't call all the centers.

"If salaries can be made comparable – and they are roughly comparable now – people may find that their money goes a little farther in the rural areas, which might be an incentive for mental health personnel to move there."

Since grants have been made to rural areas, the situation is slightly better, says Dolan. Also, a Gallup poll of four years ago revealed that a high percentage of people want to live in the rural areas and small towns. And she adds, "we are beginning to get some people who want to go to the rural areas and who are leaving the cities, but it is not such a return flow that we are having a housing shortage."

The big barrier to bringing professional people to the rural areas, says Dolan, is the poor education systems. "They don't want their children to go to the schools there. First thing a town used to build was a hotel because when the people got there they would need a place to stay. Now towns should 'beef up' their education systems. If they want professional people they should be able to recommend their schools as being of high quality, and they are not now."

Mental Health Statistics. Statistics on just how many mentally ill people there are in the country or the Intermountain states are difficult to obtain. Hospital rates are not a good indicator. In fact, they were once used to "prove" that cities are mentally unhealthy and to enforce social prejudices. Prior to the Civil War, for example, anti-abolitionists quoted studies showing that mental hospital rates among freed slaves in the North were higher than rates among rural southern slaves. They failed to notice (or mention) that in the South there were almost no beds that blacks could occupy (Srole, 1972). Still, it is amazing that half of our hospital beds are occupied by mental patients (Whitehead, 1972).

Whitehead says that it has been "estimated that at least 10 percent of our population, adults and children, has moderate to severe emotional problems which interfere with comfortable and productive living."

This same percentage holds true for Utah, says the Utah State Board of Mental Health. But only about 10 percent, or ten thousand people, received help in 1971 from public and private sources. Says Whitehead, "This leaves large numbers of people whose needs are not met and whose lives are not as happy and productive as they might be."

Both Dolan and Whitehead say that several areas of human problems such as crime or suicide can be indicators of mental illness. Whitehead says that incidence of suicide in Utah is higher than the national average and that self-inflicted deaths in teenagers and young adults may be the leading cause of death in this age group. Utah's divorce rate is also higher than the national average and the illegitimacy rate, although lower than the national average, has been significantly increasing during the past few years.

Factors in Rural Mental Illness. The Montana study by Kraenzel and Macdonald (1971) concluded that there is often a lack of purpose and disorganization in sparsely settled areas, and that can lead to mental health problems. The age of agricultural technology has removed many people from the role and status prospects agriculture can give them. Depopulation has taken away most of the other persons whom they might emulate and who would serve as role and status models. Counseling is a weak approach, say Kraenzel and Macdonald, when there is a lack of models who function appropriately; and moving away from an area, while an easy solution for outsiders to suggest, is not necessarily a constructive course of action.

Case history information in the Montana study included the farm or business owner who, seeing no future in his depopulation community, let his business be destroyed and became mentally ill. The same could very well apply to the Vietnam veteran today. Or there is the middle-aged World War II hero who had no skill that he could develop in the absence of on-the-job training. If there are more males than females in a town, what also happens to his husband-father role? A single male in a rural area can indeed be without a role. How single male adults can avoid mental illness when being "a man," especially one who is integrated into the community, is a difficult task under such circumstances.

Or the woman with as much education as her sister who migrated out, and who has more education than the typically educated male – what kind of adult job can she have in a sparsely populated area? She can marry an established farmer or business man, a potential "bum," or remain single and unemployed in a familistic society.

Conditions in sparsely populated regions are such that "residents are confronted with the immense task of purposeful role and status determination, evaluation, and invention for their own survival" (Kraenzel and Macdonald, 1971).

Education and Housing

There are two more socioeconomic factors that are important when discussing rural health. One is educational levels and can be another indicator of good or poor health in a region. *Rurality, Poverty, and Health* (U.S. Department of Agriculture, 1970) reports that those with lower amounts of education are less likely to use information about nutrition, hygiene, natal care, and so on, and that those with lower education have more days lost from work because of illness or injury. A lack of schooling can result in lower earning capacities, higher rates of unemployment, fewer trips to the dentist, higher percentage of chronic disease, and ignorance of nutrition, sanitation, and remedial health measures.

Most people today, however, receive a high school education, but there is little or no national difference in urban-rural years of school completed to twelve years. It is in the post-high school years that the metropolitan areas have the advantage. To the extent that a college education adds significantly to the average lifetime income, the real relative deficit in higher education in nonmetropolitan areas constitutes a substantial disadvantage (U.S. Congress, 1971). Only half of eligible rural, as compared to urban, young people go to college, and the higher percentage of young people in the rural areas makes this discrepancy even larger.

A study done by Erickson (1972), concerning warning signs for serious disease, found that while the percentage was not great, education levels did enhance knowledge of Intermountain Area residents. Of the general population surveyed, 57 percent knew the warning signals for cancer, 42 percent for heart disease, and 28 percent for stroke. Of college students, 65 percent were familiar with cancer signals, 49 percent with heart disease signs, and 33 percent with warning signs of stroke.

The Intermountain Region has a consistently higher median level of education than the nation when the Intermountain urban fringe (surburban) is compared with the U.S. urban fringe (suburban), and likewise for both rural areas as seen in Table 8-7. Utah and Colorado tie for the highest educated urban fringe, at 12.6 years for males and 12.5 years for females. Utah has the highest averages for rural residents, with both men and women receiving 12.3 years of education in each. National averages are 12.4 and 10.7 for males, suburban and rural respectively, and 12.3 and 11.5 for females. Consistently, however, the Intermountain suburbanites have a higher education median than do the Intermountain rural residents. The greatest difference is found among Montana males, where city students get 12.4 years of education and rural youths average 11.9 years.

Adequate housing is another important component of sound rural health, contributing not only to the well-being of the families and individuals, but helping to create a satisfying environment for the whole community. Over the past two decades, according to the *Economic and Social Conditions* (U.S. Congress, 1971), there has been considerable improvement in the housing picture in the Unites States. Although nonmetropolitan areas, with 30 percent of the population, still have 60 percent of the substandard units,[5] this figure is down from 65 percent in 1950. The number of occupied substandard units in nonmetropolitan areas has declined by 7.2 million in the last twenty years.

The congressional report states that this improvement is closely related to the reduction in the number of families with poverty level incomes and to the fact that in nonmetropolitan areas there were more new housing starts and more renovation than new households formed. During the two decades, 1950–1970, there were 10.1 million new housing units started in nonmetropolitan areas. During this same period of time, 1.2 million new households were

---

[5]Substandard housing has been defined by federal housing agencies as housing that lacked complete plumbing facilities or that had complete plumbing facilities but were rated dilapidated by census enumerators.

Table 8-7

Median Level of Education for Rural and Suburban Residents, 25 Years of Age and Older, in the Intermountain States as Compares to U.S. Men and Women

(1970)

Place/Sex	Suburban (Urban Fringe)	Rural	Difference
Colorado:			
Men	12.6	12.2	0.4
Women	12.5	12.3	0.2
Idaho:			
Men	12.5	12.1	0.4
Women	12.5	12.2	0.3
Montana:			
Men	12.4	11.9	0.5
Women	12.3	12.2	0.1
Nevada:			
Men	12.4	12.2	0.2
Women	12.4	12.3	0.1
Utah:			
Men	12.6	12.3	0.3
Women	12.5	12.3	0.2
Wyoming:			
Men	(a)	12.1	(a)
Women	(a)	12.3	(a)
United States:			
Men	12.4	10.7	0.7
Women	12.3	11.5	0.8

[a]No Wyoming SMSAs.

Source: Bureau of the Census, U.S. Department of Commerce, **Census of the Population, 1970**, vol. I, parts, 1, 7, 14, 28, 30, 46, and 52 (Washington, D.C.: U.S. Government Printing Office, 1970); Bureau of the Census, U.S. Department of Commerce, **Summary, Colorado, Idaho, Montana, Nevada, Utah, and Wyoming** (Washington, D.C.: U.S. Government Printing Office, 1973).

added in nonmetropolitan areas. Thus, the 10.1 million new housing units substantially accounted for improvement in housing, replacing 7.2 million substandard houses, providing housing for 1.2 million added households, and taking the place of 1.2 million lost by fire, demolition, or other causes.

But despite improvements, substandard houses still exist, and many can be found in the Intermountain Region, as Table 8-8 reveals, although the situation here is not as critical as in other areas of the United States. Even the region's highest percentage of rural substandard housing, which is 16.8 in Montana, is considerably better than the national average of 19.4. Yet this 16.8 percent means that almost one in every six Montana residents lives in either dilapidated houses or homes lacking some or all plumbing.

Rural housing in the Intermountain Region is consistently more substandard than urban housing. More than three times as many rural residents live in substandard homes than do urban Coloradoans, Utahns, and Nevadans, and the figure is almost as high for those living in Idaho. Montana, a state with few large cities, was high for both rural and urban substandard housing. The *Montana State Plan* (1973) estimated that of the 19,897 overcrowded housing units in Montana, 11,367 are in rural areas. Data on Wyoming were not available, but with such a high rurality it would be reasonable to assume that housing statistics there are not particularly good.

Many health problems are more likely to occur when people live in substandard homes. Lack of electricity can mean poor eyesight for those in dim houses, or poor diets contributed to by lack of refrigeration. According to *Montana State Plan* (1973):

> A number of diseases are related to inadequate housing. Many respiratory infections are related to inadequate heating or ventilation and inadequate and crowded sleeping arrangements. Gastro-intestinal diseases are casually related to crowding inadequate water and sewage disposal facilities, or the multiple use of toilet, water, sleeping and food handling facilities. Rats proliferate where environmental sanitation in the neighborhood environment is inadequate. Perhaps the major health problem associated with housing is the accidental injuries that occur in homes and that are related to conditions such as general disrepair, poor lighting, poor electrical connections, crowded conditions and substandard con-

Table 8-8

Substandard Housing in Rural and Suburban Areas of the Intermountain Region

(1970)

Type of Area	Total Year-Round Units		Number Lacking Some or All Plumbing		Number Dilapidated (with all plumbing)		Substandard Total Number		Substandard Percentage	
	Rural	Suburban	Rural	Suburban	Rural	Suburban	Rural	Suburban	Rural	Suburban
Colorado	169,459	247,804	19,926	5,714	5,694	3,529	25,620	9,243	15.1%	3.7%
Idaho	108,631	11,153	8,940	232	3,772	245	12,712	477	11.7	4.3
Montana	112,341	14,450	15,140	1,126	3,767	331	18,907	1,457	16.8	10.1
Nevada	34,291	66,217	2,630	1,029	1,134	1,346	3,764	2,375	11.0	3.6
Utah	61,620	128,505	4,489	1,169	2,058	1,918	6,547	3,087	10.6	2.4
Wyoming	45,465	—	4,959	—	1,545	—	6,504	—	14.3	—
All states in the Intermountain Region	531,807	468,129	56,084	9,270	17,970	7,369	74,054	16,639	13.9	3.6
United States	17,696,662	23,449,213	2,982,189	831,570	459,964	466,270	3,442,153	1,297,840	19.5	5.5

Source: Bureau of the Census, U.S. Department of Commerce, **Plumbing Facilities and Estimates of Dilapidated Housing, 1970** (Washington, D.C.: U.S. Government Printing Office, 1973).

struction. Nationally, these accidents affect about 25 million people in their homes each year, and constitute one-third of all non-fatal and one-fourth of all fatal injuries that occur.

Selected References

Coe, Maynard. "Making Agriculture Safe." *Journal of the Kansas State Medical Society* (February 1959).

Cohen, Julius. "The Effect of Distance on Use of Outpatient Services in a Rural Mental Health Center." *Hospital and Community Psychiatry* (March 1972).

Colorado State Division of Administrative Services. *Colorado Vital Statistics.* Denver: Department of Health. 1973.

Council on Rural Health, American Medical Association. "Priorities for Establishing a Rural Emergency Medical Services System." *Rural Health News* (February 2, 1975), no. 1.

Erickson, Donald L. "Consumer Health Education: A Rural Renaissance." *Rocky Mountain Medical Journal* (December 1972).

Ford, Thomas R. *Health and Demography in Kentucky.* Lexington: University of Kentucky Press. 1964.

Idaho State Bureau of Vital Statistics. *Annual Report, 1973.* Boise: Department of Health and Welfare. 1973.

Jones, James D.; *et al.* "Profile of the Rural Community Mental Health Center." Expanded version of paper presented at the 53d Meeting of the American Country Life Association, Kalamazoo, Michigan, July 1974.

Kraenzel, Carl F.; and Macdonald, Frances H. *Social Forces in Rural Communities of Sparsely Populated Areas.* Bozeman: Montana State University Agricultural Experiment Station. February 1971.

Montana State Bureau of Records and Statistics. *Montana Vital Statistics, 1972.* Helena: Department of Health and Environmental Science. 1972.

_________ Division of Comprehensive Health Planning. *Montana State Plan for Health.* Helena: Department of Health and Environmental Science. August 1974.

________ Highway Traffic Safety Division. "Summary of Motor Vehicle Accidents from January 1, 1974, to December 31, 1974." Helena: Department of Intergovernmental Relations. 1975.

Nevada State Office of Comprehensive Health Planning. *Preventive Health Services.* 1974.

Powers, John H., M.D. "The Hazards of Rural Living." *Surgery, Gynecology & Obstetrics* (August 1958).

Srole, Leo. "Urbanization and Mental Health: Some Reformations." *American Scientist* (September-October 1972), vol. 60.

U.S. Congress, Senate, Committee on Government Operations. *The Economic and Social Conditions of Rural America in the 1970s: Impact of Department of HEW Programs on Nonmetropolitan Areas, 1970.* 92d Cong., 1st Sess. May 1971.

U.S. Department of Agriculture. *Rurality, Poverty and Health.* Agricultural Economic Report No. 172. Washington D.C.: U.S. Department of Agriculture. February 1970.

________, Rural Development Service. *Health Services in Rural America.* Agriculture Information Bulletin No. 362. Washington, D.C.: U.S. Department of Agriculture. 1973.

U.S. Department of Health, Education, and Welfare, Health Resources Administration. *Area Resource File.* Rockville, Maryland: Division of Manpower Intelligence, Bureau of Health Resources. April 1974.

________, Public Health Service. *Patients at Federally Funded Community Mental Health Center in 1971.* Statistical Note 102. Rockville, Maryland: National Institute of Mental Health. 1974.

Utah State Department of Social Services. *Utah Health Facts.* Salt Lake City: Center for Health Statistics. May 1972.

________ Division of Health. *Utah Health Profile.* Salt Lake City: Center for Health Statistics. December 1973.

________ Division of Mental Health. *A Mental Health System for Today and Tomorrow.* Salt Lake City: Department of Social Services. April 1975.

Waller, Julian A., M.D. "Control of Accidents in Rural Areas." *Journal of the American Medical Association* (July 17, 1967), vol. 201, no. 3.

____________. "Emergency Health Services in Areas of Low Population Density." *Journal of the American Medical Association* (March 24, 1969), vol. 207, no. 12.

Whitehead, Paul L., M.D. "Cooperation for Mental Health." *Rocky Mountain Medical Journal* (March 1972).

Wyoming State Department of Health and Social Services. *Wyoming Emergency Medical Services, 1971.* Cheyenne: Division of Health and Medical Services. March 1972.

9

Models for Improved Health Care Delivery

Chapters 7 and 8 have presented many of the problems that have had impact upon the Intermountain West and that have helped to initiate improvements in rural health and health care. However, unless the information can be applied toward a practicable working solution, presenting it here will have been of little value.

This chapter offers ideas which, it is hoped, could be used, with some adaptation, to alleviate some of the problems discussed. Today, good health care *can be* and *is being* provided to rural residents in a number of ways; but it is clear that, for many, solutions completely different from the traditional "physician in resident" must be sought. In some areas, emphasis may be needed on expanded transportation and communication capabilities, part-time use of physicians and allied health workers, improvement of biomonitoring technology, use of new physician support occupations, better understanding of individual health practicies, and development of emergency care and self-help methods to ensure rural health coverage.

This chapter includes twenty health care models, the first seven of which are now in use in parts of the Intermountain Area, several being national in scope. The remainder are effective plans that have been implemented elsewhere in the United States. But all are successful and all prove that the situation is by no means hopeless.

The American Medical Association has devised a list of elements that would be included in an "ideal" rural health delivery system. All of the models presented in this chapter incorporate at least some of these aspects:

(1) Personnel
  (a) Two or more physicians representing primary physician skills; e.g., family practitioner, internist, pediatrician
  (b) Nurse, dentist, laboratory and X-ray technicians
  (c) Health aides recruited from the local community
  (d) Physician's assistant or a nurse practitioner
  (e) Public health nurse for outreach and follow-up
  (f) Social worker
  (g) Administrator and staff
  (h) Medical specialists, staff, visiting or by referral

(2) Services – one door for all economic levels
  (a) Preventive, curative, and rehabilitative, both medical and dental
  (b) Social services
  (c) Transportation to and from a clinic and to referral sources
  (d) Outreach case finding
  (e) Home care
  (f) Appropriate technology
  (g) Satellite clinics
  (h) Administrative
  (i) Evaluation and medical audit
  (j) Central records, master family records, established referral and report-back procedures
  (k) Adequate physical facilities
  (l) Emergency medical services
  (m) Nutrition

(3) Community relationships
  (a) Health council representing the total community
  (b) Community college for training aides

   (c) Medical schools for referral and source of students and residents
   (d) County health department
   (e) Medical society
   (f) Health planning agencies
   (g) Citizen health education

(4) Funding – multiple method approach
   (a) Fee for service
   (b) Prepaid or capitation
   (c) Third party
   (d) Sliding scale
   (e) Public funding for nonreimbursable services

The great variety of selections and combinations illustrates that there are many types of rural health delivery systems, and each community or group of communities looking for an answer should keep this and their own individual needs in mind. Says Gunn McKay,[1] Utah Congressman and a member of the Congressional Rural Caucus:

> The people of rural America have spent a long time coping with the doctor shortage. While many rural areas also have poor quality health care, there are many which have met their health care problems with imagination and ingenuity. It is well that any federal, state, or local assistance accommodate, and not totally replace, the solutions that rural people have devised for themselves. Health planning must always be a highly flexible arrangement, with a great deal of local involvement in the planning and consideration for the unique problems, resources and existing practices of each community.

Utah's Health Maintenance Program

A program intended to demonstrate whether significant improvement in the quality and cost of health care can be achieved by physicians through voluntary cooperative organizations of health care delivery without altering their practice settings, through use of comprehensive outpatient benefits, peer review, and efficient financing has recently begun in a rural Intermountain Area. It is the Blue Cross–Blue Shield of the Utah Health Maintenance Program which began April 1975 in Vernal and Roosevelt.

[1]Personal correspondence, June 27, 1975.

The Blue Cross–Blue Shield idea is not a new one within the organization, although this is the first such program to be established in Utah. It was originated by the Blue Shield Plan of the Wisconsin Medical Society. Their largest program has been operating in Dane County since about the beginning of 1973, and according to the Dane County Medical Society, has been exceptionally well accepted by the people there. Under this scheme, employer groups are offered the health maintenance plan or traditional Blue Cross–Blue Shield coverage. Employees and dependents choosing the health maintenance plan must also designate a primary care physician who will be responsible for all their primary care and for referral to services not provided by the physician.

Four family practice physicians in Roosevelt, operating as a group practice, and four solo family practice physicians in Vernal have agreed to provide services for the people who join the health maintenance program. However, physicians do not have to accept a set amount of members and can refuse individuals if they choose. So far, a thousand people in about 35 to forty employer groups have become members. Target goal is two thousand, with a maximum of four thousand members. Characteristics of each employer group are taken as a whole in determining monthly premiums.

One of the major features of the health maintenance plan is the grouping of several primary care physicians into a health maintenance account. The full health care premium of those members served by the physicians – minus 20 percent for administration, marketing, out-of-area benefits, and reinsurance to the physicians – will be allocated to the health maintenance account. From this account physicians will be paid a capitation amount for those persons who select them as their primary care physician.

This prepayment to the physician covers the high-volume, low-cost services such as office visits, laboratory work, X ray, and preventive care. Specific capitation amounts will depend on the type of patient the physician treats; i.e., child only, adult woman only, and so on. In addition, the primary care physician will be responsible for monitoring and approving expenditure of the pooled funds in the health maintenance account for other health care services received by his or her members, such as referral physician care, prescription drugs, hospital care, and so forth.

Participating referral care physicians are paid on a usual, customary, and reasonable fee-for-service basis directly by the health maintenance program. If a member receives care from a nonparticipating physician, he or she must pay the physician according to that doctor's own rates and will then be reimbursed by the program, but only up to a predetermined amount.

If individual members seek care on their own, i.e., not through their primary physician, the program is not obligated to make any payment except in cases of emergency. Blue Cross hospitals are expected to participate also, and will be paid on the same basis provided for in their regular Blue Cross agreement.

The referral system, says Evan Schelin,[2] director of Blue Cross–Blue Shield's Product Development, will give the primary physician more opportunity and responsibility in determining what services are required for the proper care of patients. The member won't have to look for a physician when he or she needs care. "If a person has a urinary tract problem, for example," says Schelin, "instead of the doctor saying, 'You ought to see a urologist and get that taken care of,' the doctor sees to it that the person gets an appointment with a urologist."

This commitment by the primary physician, along with a regular review by the other doctors in the health maintenance account of services he renders or arranges for, is to serve as a basis for quality and cost control. Blue Cross–Blue Shield will provide the physicians with monthly and quarterly printouts describing services rendered. This information will enable them to determine the number of office calls that they have individually provided and also the number of referrals generated and hospital days created. In this way the physicians share in the responsibility and give mutual support to one another in determining the appropriateness and cost of services furnished to their members.

At the end of each operational year, the health maintenance account will be closed and the financial status examined. If there is a surplus, the physician will retain one-third, Blue Cross–Blue Shield will keep one-third for the members, and the hospitals will get the final third. If there is a deficit, Blue Cross–Blue Shield will absorb full losses. In addition, during the first year the capitation payment will be guaranteed at 90 percent of what the physicians would have earned had they been functioning on a fee-for-service basis.

---

[2]Telephone interview, March 10, 1975.

Schelin feels that the plan is an advantage for both doctors and the subscribers involved. "We want to provide the members with comprehensive services and to see if in providing those services there can be a voluntary system that provides for efficient financing and improves the cost and quality of health care." He fells that such a system will benefit the consumer because their doctors accept the responsibility for the management of their health and voluntarily submit to a review by their colleagues that extends to both the appropriateness of the service as well as the dollars spent. The end result should be high-quality and low-cost medical care.

It benefits the physician in that there is reduced paperwork and thus reduced office expenses, he says. When a physician renders a service covered under capitation he doesn't have to file a claim and Blue Cross–Blue Shield doesn't have to process it. Instead, the doctors simply check a block on a preprinted form to note services rendered. This information is sent to Blue Cross–Blue Shield for statistical data. "Additionally," says Schelin, "it removes many of the traditional third party restraints and administrative hassles. The physician is going to be free to render or order whatever care he deems appropriate and in the setting of his choice. The health maintenance program isn't going to try and second-guess him as to whether the hospitalization was necessary or whether the diagnosis really justified his ordering a particular lab or X-ray service. We want that kind of dialog to be among the physicians in the health maintenance account, not between the plan and the physician."

While the plan is already operating, it is by no means finalized. Certain aspects are still under debate, and approval as a health maintenance organization has not been received, although Schelin feels this should come soon. Future plans are for the health maintenance program to expand to several other rural areas in the state, and then to one populous Wasatch Front area before the end of the year.

Originally, Blue Cross–Blue Shield had hoped to establish a health maintenance program in the Salt Lake area, but physicians there had too many "unresolved questions on how it would affect their practice and particularly about this mode of payment," said Schelin. "Several of the doctors in Vernal and Roosevelt have the same concerns, but they were willing to give it a try on a limited basis."

Group Practice in Colorado[3]

Kremmling Clinic. Dr. Ernest Ceriani has been practicing medicine for 27 years to the several thousand people who live in the mountainous ranching country around Kremmling, Colorado. When he began, Kremmling had four hundred to five hundred people and an outreach of fifteen hundred people. Today, Grand County has a population of 5,800 and Kremmling itself has a thousand inhabitants. The population is basically homogeneous, white, middle class by rural standards, with 26.4 percent of the population earning between $5,000 to $7,999 in 1971. There is a low incidence of welfare recipients according to Dr. Ceriani. At least a third of the population is 65 years or older.

Ceriani fits the model of the rural boy returning to practice medicine in the rural setting. He began as a solo practitioner but after five years began recruiting for another doctor in order to set up a group. He is convinced that group practice "makes more sense all the time." He has no clear-cut format for such a service, but unlike its urban counterpart – a collection of specialists – the rural group would amount to a nucleus of primary care physicians. The group could provide the desired professional interdependence for its members and alleviate such common objections to solo rural practice as too rigorous a work schedule with no time off and the lack of colleagues with whom to discuss problems. In addition, Dr. Ceriani envisions that a group could serve as a referral or guidance center for several "satellite" medical practitioners – ranging perhaps from a family physician to a highly trained paramedic – dotted about the surrounding area.

At present, the Kremmling Clinic consists of a clinic building and the Kremmling Hospital, a "drawing card" to attract physicians to the rural area. Literature shows that those rural areas with an existing hospital have a better chance of attracting physicians than an area without a hospital.

The Kremmling Clinic is staffed by Dr. Ceriani and his two young associates. A fourth physician, an experienced practitioner, left Kremmling to take over a vacant clinic in a nearby town, a facility that is now, in effect, a satellite practice.

---

[3]Taken from a paper by Richard Spears, Sarah Bowman, Hilda Grey, and John Kralewski, Ph.D.

The hospital has twenty beds and, according to Ceriani, it's usually "a full house.... It's always musical beds around there. When I left [to come to a rural health conference where he was interviewed] there was a variety of patients from an 86-year-old woman with heart disease who had broken her angle to an O.B."

Nursing recruitment for the hospital is satisfactory – one RN and one aide for each of the three shifts for twenty beds. Dr. Ceriani recalled that at one time, "two nurses worked twelve-hour shifts, seven days a week, for two years." Now the nurses are paid salaries commensurate with Denver salaries and get incentives for continuing and in-service education. However, there is not a pool of nurses from which to recruit; if there is a storm and the night nurse is snowed in, Dr. Ceriani himself has been known to "pull a shift."

Dr. Ceriani sees use of the paramedic as a great help in his health care delivery plan. They are professionals who could be "a vital force" in rural medicine by caring for "a third to a half of the 95 percent of ailments that patients bring through the front door," says Dr. Ceriani. He would like to use those individuals who do not want or need an M.D. degree but feel that health care is their field. Such a career could be personally – and monetarily – satisfying, says Ceriani, although "there are other professionals that can offer more money than what we make." At present the Kremmling group does not have a paramedic but plans to soon.

Patients are on a fee-for-service basis, and Dr. Ceriani's group takes Medicare and Medicaid. Group members get 50 percent of what they put on the book and can become a partner after one year's service. He was not sure how much the group had to "write off" each year.

On an average day, from forty to sixty patients are seen. "It used to be I had to see that many alone," he said, "but now there are three of us to divide up the work." Nearly 95 percent of the patients are treated at Kremmling Clinic and Hospital. The group uses backup help from Denver, especially for complicated procedures such as orthopedics.

When Ceriani began his recruitment efforts, the usual routes were essentially a failure. He estimates that he has spent between \$3,000 and \$5,000 over the years advertising in the *Journal of the American Medical Association* and other medical journals. "This price also includes a series of abortive collect phone calls which never materialized into one new group member." He feels that the best method is to try to recruit people out of their rotating internship or family practice residency and not put too much pressure on them. "You have to be flexible because these young chaps are searching for something and they don't want to make a long-term commitment," he said, adding that many would like a rural group practice setting but want to try it first. Also, some young doctors want to do general practice with the option of returning for additional training such as internal medicine or general surgery. "They essentially don't want to do solo practice but also don't want a long-term commitment."

An M.D.'s wife also influences his decision to go into a group practice in the rural areas, believes Ceriani. As the children start to get older, the wives feel that they (children) need the cultural advantages of the city and pressure husbands to leave the rural practice. A woman who has many self-sufficient interests appears to fare better than a woman who is dependent on the community to provide her social life. This factor in recruitment of doctors to the rural area is often overlooked, Dr. Ceriani feels.

Finally, Dr. Ceriani says that there are no major answers to the manpower or distribution problems, only questions. "If there is a secret to recruitment, it's in the area of the multi-doctor concept."

Summit County Groups. The Summit Medical Center is located in the town of Frisco in Summit County, Colorado. Summit County has a population of 3,800 people, with 48.8 percent earning over $10,000 a year. There has been a recent increase in permanent county residents as a result of the Eisenhower Tunnel project, plus a large number of people who enter the area each year for resort and recreational purposes.

Dr. John Swearingen heads a group of four physicians at the Summit Medical Center, and he and one other doctor work only part time during peak times like the winter ski season. Another member is Dr. A. Lewis, another rural boy who has returned to practice medicine in the country. After finishing the family practice residency at Colorado General Hospital, he had planned to return to rural Virginia where both his father and grandfather had practiced medicine. At that time (about two and a half years ago) Swearingen contacted Lewis, asking if he (Lewis) would be interested in working in a group that Swearingen was considering building. This method of contacting family practice residents was Swearingen's method of recruiting group members.

The clinic itself has been in existence since 1972, and Dr. Lewis sees the emergency room as one of its fine points, especially during the ski season, as the clinic serves Keystone, Copper Mountain, Breckenridge, and Arapahoe Basin ski areas. On an average ski weekend, there are often up to ten people at a time on the stretcher and a busy day brings in, on the average, 55 people. "During the peak of the ski season the emergency room can accommodate the crowds beautifully," says Lewis.

Most ski injuries seen are skull lacerations and broken tibiae, depending on the condition of the snow. Lacerations are seen when it is icy and more tears occur when the snow is wet, says Dr. Lewis. "I still ski, but very carefully, and after seeing all the injuries, I almost don't enjoy downhill skiing anymore."

Prior to 1972, the only other medical providers in nearby Dillon were a foreign M.D. and an osteopath. When the Summit group opened, most of the patients were taken away from the other M.D., and county records show she had unkind things to say about Dr. Swearingen's group. At present she is practicing on an Indian reservation and planning to return to Dillon, but Lewis does not anticipate any competition.

Dr. Lewis estimates that he and the other full-time physician see approximately thirty patients each on an average day. Swearingen and the other part-time doctor each see seventeen to twenty a day, five days a week, including patients in the clinic and in the emergency room. This staffing pattern seems adequate even for the peak season, and the only inadequacy in Dr. Lewis' mind is the lack of holding beds.

Concerning the family of a rural doctor and how they adjust to the rural setting, a variety of patterns can be seen in the Summit group. Dr. Lewis' wife grew up in the city, has had a rather difficult adjustment to the rural area, and misses the social contacts of the city. Also, he says she feels very "hemmed in" with a two-year-old and expecting a second child (at time of interview). This has put a lot of pressure on Dr. Lewis but they both are working toward solutions. The Lewises have discussed the possibility of her attending Colorado Women's College in Denver a few days a week, since her parents live in Denver and they could care for the children. Dr. Sudwicks, the other full-time member, and his wife are from rural Idaho and, at the time of the interview, had two young children. They seem to like the recreation facilities; Mrs. Sudwicks in particular likes rural life and has become involved in many local functions. However, they are concerned about the education component in Summit County, and the fact that few children attend college. Well-paying construction work is readily available in and around Summit County; many adolescents do not see the need for higher education. The fourth member of the group is a bachelor.

Two RNs are connected with the office, one working two days a week and the other three days a week. Dr. Swearingen has hired a former medic from the Army and has trained him to do X rays and casting as well as to serve as an emergency room nurse. A laboratory technician does routine tests, but complicated ones must be sent to Upjohn Laboratories.

The clinic does not have its own ambulance and uses the Summit County's ambulance for emergency service to Denver. An emergency medical trainee handled many of the complicated cases in 1973 but did not stay on, placing a terrible burden on the volunteer drivers. Both doctors have accompanied patients to Denver because they were afraid to let them go alone. Emergency personnel are being recruited, especially for the busy ski season. West Summit group patients are sent to Lutheran or Colorado General Hospitals depending on the patient's ability to pay.

Two physician assistants have been used; one was very successful and the other was not. A child health associate was well received, and the parents were pleased with her work, but an adult nurse practitioner had a different experience. Patients complained about their bills after having seen the practitioner, and Dr. Lewis admitted that perhaps the other doctors did not attempt to socialize the patients about the role of the nurse practitioner.

A county public health nurse provides family planning service, nutrition counseling, and immunization programs. Specialty care is given by the Gottesfilds, an obstetric-gynecology group who come from Denver once a week and follow up on a few patients, and Dr. Swearingen who is an orthopedist. Two dentists in Dillon provide dental care, and a physical therapist works part time with patients who need rehabilitation services. The Summit group also takes advantage of the wefare officer who helps with patients needing welfare or children living in unhealthy circumstances.

There are no outside administrators and Swearingen makes most of these decisions. Informal information sharing is done among the doctors. For example, if one of the group goes to a medical meeting, he makes a report to the other members upon his return. Chart review is done at the end of the day, also on an informal basis.

Most work is done by fee for service. The patient who has Blue Cross and Blue Shield can seek necessary help from the group's secretary on filling out forms. Sliding scale has been used on occasions and local pharmacists will give these patients a reduced rate if the doctors put a red mark on the prescription. The clinic receives some money for VD control and family planning from the Colorado State Department of Health. All the gamma globulin used for hepatitis can be obtained free from the state health department. The medical group is salaried, including Dr. Swearingen.

Yampa Valley Family Health Center. Steamboat Springs has a population of 2,271, with Routt County having a population of 6,344. The income breakdown for this county shows that 23.4 percent of the population makes $5,000 to $7,999 annually, and 20.7 percent makes more than $10,000. The major sources of income include agriculture, mining, and more recently, ski and other recreation and sports facilities.

Yampa Valley Family Health Center was established in 1972 and in 1975 had two family practice physicians, two registered nurses, one office assistant and a part-time counselor who worked with mental health problems. A nutritionist consultant and a medical technologist came in on a regular basis. The group also uses the local public health nurse, as well as welfare workers when necessary.

The services the group provides are primarily broadly based ambulatory and preventive care. Well-baby and basic pediatric care compose a large portion of their time. The doctors encourage breast feeding and do as much patient teaching as they can during their visits with patients. Trauma care also composes a large part of their practice.

A problem-oriented record system is used, and the doctors are very conscientious about evaluation of patient care and medical audit. The Denver-based Rural Health Care Association has assisted with recruitment and other problems since 1972.

Steamboat Springs is part of a functioning Comprehensive Health Planning Commission, but it is not yet effectual on the local level. There is a community college, but it has no training for medical personnel, such as aides. There is no county health department, a citizen's health education program is sorely lacking, and even schools view health education with suspicion. Some of the family practice residents from Colorado General Hospital do rotate in Steamboat Springs.

Funding is primarily a fee-for-service mechanism with some third party payers but no prepaid groups. The medical group members are salaried and after one year are entitled to a full partnership in the corporation.

Dr. Bruce Amondson and his group members "put together a group before they put together a location – which in itself is different." The three people involved were Amondson, Dr. Hoffman, who was Dr. Amondson's associate from medical school, and Mr. Peterson, a health care administrator.

When Amondson left the family practice residency at the University of Oklahoma, the Amondson family traveled for two months looking for potential communities. "We had defined some guidelines in terms of where we wanted to live. We looked at the West and at communities primarily with a population under 10,000." With that in mind, they spent time in several communities trying to determine the need for health care. They spoke with providers and consumers, including newspaper editors, businessmen, physicians, hospital administrators, and bankers, trying to get some idea of what these people saw as the medical care needs in that region and the potential for developing a system of health care versus the fragmentation that exists in too many communities. It was narrowed down to four communities: one in Idaho, one in Minnesota, one in Wyoming, and Steamboat Springs, at the request of Dr. Kralewski, a associate professor at the University of Colorado Medical Center and director of the Division of Health Administration, who was a friend of Mr. Peterson.

A series of criteria, both professional and personal, had been developed, including size of the community, presence of a college, quality of the school system, availability of recreation, presence of a hospital, need for physicians, and the existing medical community. Each member of the group rated the four communities, and Steamboat Springs was selected. Amondson says that he would do it this way again; however, had they spent more time in Steamboat Springs, they might not have gone there in view of the rapid growth, rapid recreation changes, and some of the devisiveness going on in the medical community. Amondson says he would recommend that doctors trying to recruit other doctors for a group practice look at both the community health needs and what the community has to offer, then mesh these with the doctor's goals, including the goal of developing a system of family-oriented health care.

When Amondson's group arrived in Steamboat Springs, there were two solo physicians searching for a third doctor for the town, but the arrival of a group was really the genesis of problems which are not yet washed away. The family practice group was just out of training and wanting changes to occur. What resulted was a kind of a "future shock" reaction in the health community, as both the doctors and the nurses were all accustomed to doing things in a patterned way. Now, not only was there more for the nurses to do, but more things were demanded of them. A meeting was held that almost evolved into a lynch mob mentality based on resistance to change and the villification of the change agents. Simply, the psychological discomfort when change was occurring at a rapid rate was the problem. The hospital (of twenty beds, not Joint Commission approved but state health department licensed) became the focus of the problem in the medical community. Ironically, the original physicians recruited a third physician who was in internal medicine and who was making demands on the hospital as well.

Both Peterson and Hoffman left within a year of their arrival. Now there are two new members of the medical group, but how to keep doctors is still an unresolved problem in Dr. Amondson's mind. One of the new group members, a competent family practice practitioner, is leaving to take his surgical residency shortly. Dr. Amondson feels that this problem of retaining group members has to do with the continued problem of viability of family group practice as it relates to physician satisfaction. This member is well trained and very competent, but the frustration of dealing with some types of problems – the psychosocial problems for one – is frustrating to him, especially having to continually reaffirm credibility with patients.

Currently a general surgeon and an orthopedist are in the community. The general practitioners originally in the area do some general surgery and do it well. The general surgeon is currently doing itinerant surgery in Rangely where there is a small community hospital, but post-operative care is a problem. He does the surgery but leaves the post-operative care to the local practitioner. This policy of itinerant surgery is not accepted by the American College of Surgeons, but is being accepted by the people in the rural communities as it enables the patient to stay at home for care.

There are doctors who flee to the rural communities because of problems such as alcoholism or feelings of inadequacy. Medical doctors with severe sociopathic problems want to avoid the high visibility of the urban centers and flee to the rural areas and perform an inferior quality of health care delivery. "People in rural areas have a right to good health care and don't want to settle for incompetence," Amondson said. "We need assistance from consultants in order to help us do as much as we can competently do in the community."

This could help change what Amondson calls a "warehouse mentality, a mentality that makes hospital personnel ask 'When do we ship the patient?" . . . The pattern of care that developed was that you didn't improve your medical competence for handling the situation, you simply shipped them out. This made the providers feel comfortable because they had no complications to deal with. This has changed a tremendous amount in three years, and the first question asked now is not 'when do we ship' but 'how do we care for' the patient."

One of the most important devices in continuing education has been a carefully worked out network of consultation basically from Denver. An orthopedic surgeon came to teach the community on-site consultation cooperation. "We would schedule patients every three weeks or so and he would come out and work with the group, teaching them the needed procedures in acute orthopedic care," said Dr. Amondson. Out of this interrelationship came a conference at St. Joseph's Hospital, a co-equal relationship between family practice and orthopedic surgeons in a co-equal dialog. "For example, if someone came into Denver with a complicated fracture, the orthopedist knew what our group capabilities were and he felt confident about sending patients home to Steamboat, knowing the patient would get good care from us." This co-equal medical relationship will discourage more general practice people from leaving their profession for a specialty if this respect between generalist and specialist can become well established.

Conclusions. Physicians choosing to practice in a rural area are frequently looking for more than a place to practice medicine. Communities recruiting physicians may overlook this self-selection that causes only some doctors to consider a rural location.

Dr. Ceriani is an example of the rural boy returning to practice in the rural area. He suggested giving young physicians wide flexibility and options for leaving if they desire to do so. He does not want to lose members constantly, but feels that the new breed of physicians do not want long-term commitments. He can assure new physicians that they will be completely in charge of their patients and will have expert opinions available, if needed, from backup personnel in Denver.

The need to be a "big fish in a little pond" can be fulfilled in a group practice in the rural area. Also, the doctor can cultivate other interests in a group practice and still earn an adequate salary, such as Dr. Ceriani's group, where 50 percent of what the physician puts on the books can be earned. Also, Dr. Ceriani pointed out the need for spouses of physicians in a rural community to be fairly self-sufficient people who can entertain themselves without big city stimulation.

Dr. Lewis pointed out that one method of recruiting group physicians was to contact people finishing a family practice residency. He also stated there is a need for holding beds or a community hospital in order to follow patients who need more than primary care, and pointed out the importance of training emergency medical personel so that patients could be safely sent to Denver.

Dr. Amondson suggested gathering a compatible group together before selecting a location, then setting up criteria, and limiting the search to one geographical area with a certain population. He discussed candid feelings about rural people deserving good medical care, and suggested more co-equal medical relationships should be pondered carefully by generalist and specialists alike.

The problems of small communities which make them unattractive have been stated many times. A strong sense of community independence and pride, often accompanied by a fight for economic survival, has given rise to many traditional rivalries, including the medical care system. A community with its own school and hospital, its own physicians, and its own pharmacy, tries to keep it that way, regardless of duplication and inefficiency, because these resources bring more people into the community to patronize the local businesses. Any removal of these resources will be opposed strongly by the business community. Small communities often had a difficult time acquiring what they do have; thus they are most reluctant to risk losing a person or a service, even if the person or service is unsatisfactory. A community is hesitant to confront an alcoholic physician in fear of losing even a dangerous, incompetent physician, for it could mean being totally without medical resources. Only intensive education by someone with a clear plan and the confidence to fulfill it can alleviate these fears and respond to the problems posed.

Health Systems Research Institute

The Health Systems Research Institute began in 1973 as a rural health care project of the federaly funded Intermountain Regional Medical Program in Salt Lake City, Utah. Since then, it has expanded and developed to become an independent, nonprofit organization delivering health care to rural communities in the Intermountain, Western Plains, and Pacific states. Specifically the Institute is delivering organized health care to Battle Mountain, Austin, and Hawthorne, Nevada; Yellowstone National Park, Harlowton, and Cut Bank, Montana; Yuma County, Arizona; Odessa, Washington, and Rawlins, Wyoming. A dozen or more additional communities are being negotiated with at any given time, says Dort Tikker, the Institute's president.

At the request of any community needing help, the Institute will make an in-depth analysis of the community's health care needs and resources. Based on the results of this profile, a proposal is prepared and presented outlining a health care plan, complete with costs and conditions for implementation. This proposal is negotiable, but once agreement is reached, it amounts to a binding, legal contract whereby the Institute assumes all responsibility for the recruitment and placement of a physician and the medical care system, with the community agreeing to pay a monthly fee for these stipulated services. The first practical test of the plan came in Battle Mountain, Lander County, Nevada, in 1974.

The financial basis for the system is a "reimbursable contract," whereby all money collected by the Health Systems Research Institute for medical services rendered are returned to that community. In other words, the community's contracting authority, which in the Battle Mountain example is the county commission, pays the Institute in advance for the contracted services (say, $12,000 per month, as an example). The Institute's physician then charges his patients the customary fee and collects in the usual manner. All such collections are then returned to the contracting authority; that is, the county commissioners.

If collections are less than the theoretical $12,000 per month, the county must absorb the deficit. If collections are more than $12,000, the county still gets every penny and may actually make money on its contract. Battle Mountain was realizing about 118 percent of its contract costs as of February 1975. Until then, the county experienced a monthly deficit (as is expected during the earlier months of any contract). The Institute's studies indicated that it would normally require one year before the break-even point for a contract was reached, but less than one year has been required in Battle Mountain.

What does Battle Mountain's physician, Dr. Minthorne D. Norton, think of the Health Systems Research Institute? "It's good," he says. "I was looking for a feasible way to practice rural medicine and this seems to be it. The toughest thing for the Institute will be to find physicians who can produce enough income to reimburse the contract. An Institute doctor has got to realize that this is a business as well as a practice, and he needs to be something of a businessman himself. He's got to get involved in the community – make friends – for the Institute as well as himself."

In addition to providing good medical care, the Health Systems Research Institute claims that its system has a substantial, positive impact on a client community's economy. Tikker, the Institute's president, explained that an Institute-sponsored community health care program not only keeps medical care dollars at home for the community but attracts additional dollars from outside. Institute physicians, clinic and hospital workers, and other employees all contribute to the local economy, and increased use of community resources, such as the hospital and clinic, means that fewer, if any, tax-support dollars are required to keep the facilities functioning.

One of the latest developments in the Institute's apparently successful program is the close and comprehensive medical backup relationship with the University of Utah Medical Center's prestigious Departments of Surgery, Internal Medicine, and Pediatrics. Specialists from these areas make regular visits to communities in the Institute's domain to assist and consult with the Institute physician and to manage special cases. When indicated, difficult or critical cases are transported to the Utah Medical Center for intensive and specialized diagnosis and care.

Dr. Frank Moody, surgeon and chairman of the Utah Medical Center's Department of Surgery, praised the partnership arrangement, saying, "We are delighted to be able to provide backup to your [Institute] physicians with our most senior people, the very best we have to offer in surgical services. This is a tremendous contribution to health care in rural areas and is consistent with our goal to provide for individuals wherever they live the very best specialty surgical care. If health care is a right – which is what we preach – it has to be that way."

Dr. Kenneth F. Maclean, a member of the Nevada State Board of Medical Examiners, also had high praise for the Health Systems Research Institute, noting: "After twenty-five years of service with the Board of Medical Examiners, and having been faced with almost insurmountable problems of providing physician care in rural Nevada counties, it is my feeling that [the Institute] has come up with the only practical, sensible solution to the problem of keeping doctors in rural areas."

Medex and Nurse Practitioners

Nonphysician primary medical care personnel whose presence can help alleviate health care problems in medically deprived areas, including rural areas, are becoming more common in the Intermountain Region. These trained individuals go by a variety of names: adult health practitioners, family nurse practitioners, women's health care practitioners, geriatric nurse practitioners, and public health nurses who function as nurse practitioners (Anderson *et al.*, 1972).

Anderson and his colleagues chose the term "nurse practitioner" to refer to a

> . . . professional nurse with a diploma, and associate degree or a baccalaureate degree who has received additional preparation in the expanded role to provide primary health care. . . .

> These nurses have been prepared to perform physical examinations, record personal health histories, initiate preventive screening and diagnostic procedures, coordinate health care needs, provide patient, family, and community health teaching and guidance, perform minor surgical procedures, and institute minor emergency procedures. They can also decide when to refer the case to a physician, and may collaborate with the physician in patient management.

Anderson *et al.* used the term "physician assistant" to refer to a "skilled person qualified by academic and practical on-the-job training to provide patient services under the supervision and direction of a licensed physician, who is responsible for the performance of that assistant." Physician assistants in Utah, Montana, Wyoming, and Idaho include child health associates, physician assistants, physician associates, and Medex (explained subsequently). According to Anderson and his co-authors:

> The functions they perform are similar to those ... [of] nurse practitioners. Since nurse practitioners are covered by different legal statutes from physician assistants, their practices can be, and often are, less supervised than those of physician assistants.

Two primary care personnel training programs in the Intermountain Region are at the University of Utah, where its Medical Center trains practitioners in its Medex Program and the School of Nursing trains them in its Family Nurse Practitioner Program.

The Medex. Medex – whose name derives from the first letters in the French term *medicien extension*, meaning physician's extension – takes advantage of people already highly trained, such as an ex-military medical corpsman with a minimum of three years of high-quality medical training and experience, including some independent duty, or an individual with equivalent training and experience in a civilian setting, such as a registered nurse. These persons are further educated and sent to medically underserved areas to assist overworked physicians, many of whom are in rural areas and almost all in family practice settings.

The Utah Medex Program began in June 1971 and is sponsored by the University of Utah College of Medicine's Department of Family and Community Medicine and the Utah State Medical Society. Eight other Medex programs are under way in the United

States, including one at the University of Washington, which originated the plan in September 1969.

The Medex performs specified tasks that usually have been in the sole domain of the physician, although these jobs do not require the extensive education of an M.D. During the one-year Medex training period, five months are spent learning clinical skills that previous training has not included, such as (in the case of former military personnel), the common ailments of women and children. Seven months are then spent with a physician preceptor where the Medex refines these skills and further develops ones that he or she will need in a particular practice setting.

By March 1975, the Utah Medex Program had placed seventy trainees and graduates, 65 of whom are in Utah, Arizona, Idaho, Montana, Wyoming, Colorado, and New Mexico.

Between twelve thousand and fifteen thousand applications are received for each University of Utah Medex class, according to William Wilson,[4] deputy director of the program. These are reviewed and about a hundred people are interviewed by telephone. Approximately thirty are then invited to Salt Lake City for a weekend of interviews with the staff, clinical faculty, physician-preceptors, and Medex graduates and trainees.

The physician preceptor's role in the initial selection process helps ensure physician-Medex compatibility, says Wilson, an important factor since the physician is eventually to hire the Medex. This compatibility is further ensured when trainees and their spouses spend one day early in their training with each preceptor in his or her town. Preceptors and trainees rate each other; those signifying a high mutual interest are matched. "Eighty percent of our original matches are still intact," says Wilson.

Preceptors, too, go through a thorough selection process. Names of interested doctors are received through recommendations by other preceptors, Medex graduates, state medical associations, and other health agencies. These doctors are then contacted and visited on site by Medex staff members. The program is explained, the doctor's need for an assistant is assessed, and it is determined if the physician's facilities are adequate for training and eventually hiring the Medex.

---

[4]Personal interview, February 11, 1975.

Both patient and physician satisfaction with Medex graduates has been high, says Wilson. "For our first three classes, patient satisfaction was rated at about ninety-seven percent," he said. "As for the doctors, most of them who have a Medex wouldn't practice without one now. It is awfully nice to have someone around to help. Face it – some of primary care is boring. You can only do so many sore throats and school physicals. But the Medex likes that – that's his bailiwick. Having a Medex around enables the doctor to spend more time with the more difficult cases."

A 1973 study of Medex preceptors, done by the university's Department of Family and Community Medicine, showed that while a candidate is still in training, using him or her as an assistant can release seven hours of the doctor's time, sufficient to see 42 additional patients or an annual increase in patient load of 10 to 42 percent.

"It makes his practice more fun, too," says Wilson. "The Medexes are young and want to learn – they are always stimulating the physician and the doctors enjoy the teaching process. And it gives the doctors someone to talk with about medicine who knows what he's talking about." And he adds, "It also gives some physicians time to get away for continuing education courses that they otherwise might miss because, without their GP, the community is completely without medical care."

John Steele has been a Medex with the Dubois Health Services in rural Dubois (population, eight hundred), Wyoming, since he graduated from Utah's program in January 1974. Originally from small Shadyside, Ohio, he found out about Medex through Intermountain Regional Medical Program literature and during one of his vacations that he's been spending in Dubois for the past ten years.

Asked what his main job as a Medex is, Steele quickly answered, "I see the patients."[5] This includes almost everything, he says, from appointments to walk-ins, to acute and chronic illnesses. "I see everything that comes through the door." Plus a few that don't come through the door. "There are a lot of older people that I regularly visit at home, and there are situations where I'm called out at night – coronary problems, respiratory problems and so on – all the things in a normal country doc situation."

---

[5]Telephone interview, March 10, 1975.

The Dubois Health Services provides the only medical care around for eight miles, he says, and Steele covers about 260 miles of road when it comes to taking care of trauma cases. "In the summer the population here swells to twelve to fifteen thousand during the hunting season. I see my share of gunshot wounds and all trauma that goes with them. It's really hard to say just how many I see; probably two or three, and that's a lot."

Medex Steele is happy with his job. "I like the communication, the challenge of the situation and the personal satisfaction that comes from resolving a patient's illness. I don't have any dislikes about what I do — some things scare me, but that's hardly a dislike."

The Nurse Practitioner. The University of Utah School of Nursing's Family Nurse Practitioner Program began in March 1973 and has graduated three classes. Another class started in September 1975. According to the class syllabus:

> The purpose of the program is to prepare generalist practitioners who will work collaboratively with physicians, be prepared to make independent judgments and to assume responsibility for providing primary health care to individuals and to families. The family nurse practitioner will be prepared to obtain health histories, perform physical examinations, initiate preventive screening and diagnostic procedures, coordinate health care needs and make appropriate referrals and provide health instruction, counseling, and guidance.

The first class, which was funded by the Intermountain Regional Medical Program, was a pilot project which graduated thirteen nurse practitioners. The remaining four classes were funded by the Division of Nursing of the U.S. Department of Health, Education, and Welfare under a contract to graduate 55 nurse practitioners. The contract expired on June 30, 1976. Additional funds may be found to continue the program, but plans are being made and in fact already being used to incorporate nurse practitioner training into regular undergraduate and graduate nursing programs, says Sue Huether,[6] project director.

Trainees, who must be at least a two-year RN and have at least two years' experience, go through a twelve-month program, with three months at the university where they have nine weeks

[6]Personal interview, June 10, 1975.

of classroom instruction at the medical center and three weeks of clinical rotation throughout the Salt Lake Valley with various specialists and at hospitals.

Another month is spent in independent study. During this time, the nurses study a specialty chosen according to the needs of the community they will work in. "For instance, medical needs at the Intermountain Indian School would be different than they would be in Nephi," the project director says.

At the completion of this phase, the nurse practitioner begins a preceptorship period spent under the guidance of her physician-preceptor. Unlike the Medex Program, nurse practitioners are responsible for finding their own preceptors, most often physicians with whom they have already worked. "She is usually from that community in the first place," says Huether, "and she and the physician have decided that she should assume more responsibility."

Traditional programs in the past have taught the nurse physical assessment skills, says Huether, adding that it was thought this should be a task only for the physician. While doctors were taught more about pathology in the assessment, nurses were taught to take a history of how the patient was coping with the problem. Now the nurses are learning more about the pathology concerned with the assessment, particularly the use of technical skill related to the use of instruments.

Says Huether, "The principal objective of the nurse practitioner is to assist the consumer of health care in maintaining, regaining, or attaining a high level of health and to assist him in being independent in his health-seeking behavior, so that he will know when he should seek out health care and when he should be able to manage the situation himself.

"The nurse practitioner does a lot of teaching in relation to that. The physician may diagnose the disease – diabetes, for example – and the nurse practitioner teaches the patient how to live with it. She teaches and helps the patient to cope as a way of maintaining health." She adds, "It is not her role to replace the physician. Her role is to meet unmet health care needs that neither the physician nor the regular nurse, with her training, can meet."

Individual nurse practitioners may have their own patients that make appointments with them, or they may work with the physician. They may do routine physical examinations, case histories, and follow up and evaluation. Each setting is unique and varies according to the resources in the community.

In most cases a physician is readily available to the nurse practitioner. "We prefer that she is in a support system," says Huether. "No one can deliver health care alone. We like them to have a doctor with them, just as a doctor likes to have a nurse in his office.

"If the physician [the nurse practitioner is with] is a general practitioner, she will see a variety of cases representing the life cycle, from the infant to the elderly. Or if she is with a specialist, she will see more specialized cases. She might handle a component of a physician's practice. She might manage all the prenatal cases, or all the infant care. She could do health maintenance, such as teach classes for diabetics on diet, exercise, and so on.

"She might also take care of the elderly for their chronic diseases for which there are no cures, but which need monitoring. Physicians hate to go to nursing homes because there is no cure for the people there. But in terms of developing plans to promote comfort, the nurse practitioner has a lot to offer. Her work in the nursing home can give the doctor more time for the more acute conditions that require a physician's skill."

Most of Utah's nurse practitioner graduates are in the rural areas, according to Ida Bickle,[7] former project director. Of the thirteen members in the first class, seven are in the almost entirely rural areas of Pierce, Rexburg, and Aberdeen (Idaho), Eagle (Colorado), and Draggerton, Escalante, and Castleton (Utah), although the Escalante nurse has not found a preceptor and therefore has not been certified as of this writing. The rest of the class works with the Mountain States Regional Medical Program in Boise, the Idaho State University Health Service in Pocatello, the Veterans Administration Hospital in Grand Junction (Colorado), the Wasatch County Hospital in Heber City (Utah), and Salt Lake City's Multi-Purpose Medical Center Clinic.

The second class started in September 1974 and returned in December 1975 to their home practices. Two are currently in Provo (Utah) and will later be placed in rural areas by LDS (Mormon) hospitals. Others are with Hill Air Force Base in Dugway (Utah), the Veterans Administration Hospital in Grand Junction (Colorado), the Indian Health Service in Roosevelt (Utah), Magic Valley

---

[7]Personal interview, February 7, 1975.

Memorial Hospital in Twin Falls (Idaho), the Holy Cross Hospital in Salt Lake City, and rural areas of Stanley (Idaho) and Fallon and Overton (Nevada). While the majority of these nurse practitioner graduates works in close contact with physicians, a few practice in geographic isolation, with the telephone as their most frequent method for communicating with their M.D.

In Stanley, Idaho, for example, nurse practitioner Marie Osborn is 65 miles away from the nearest doctor and 75 miles from her preceptors in Hailey, Idaho. She gives primary care and emergency treatment to the town's 47 year-round residents and also to the more than one million people that pass through Stanley between Memorial Day and the end of the hunting season, at the Salmon River Emergency Clinic.

Osborn didn't live in Stanley when she became involved as the town's health care provider. In fact, she had been away from the nursing profession for eighteen years while she raised her five children. But she had camped in the area and, like many others, was attracted to its beauty.

"There was a series of small accidents that I was asked to help with because people knew I was a nurse," said Osborn.[8] "Then there was a really bad accident involving four teenagers and they were seriously injured. All we had to work with were some first aid kits from the forest service, and I'd been out of it [nursing] for too long to really take care of the situation. But the worst part was that it took an ambulance two and a half hours to get here."

A short time later, Osborn and her husband hosted the Lieutenant Governor's Conference, where the head of the Idaho State Hospital Association happened to be in attendance. After Osborn mentioned her concern to him, he put a man from his staff on the situation. "And," says Osborn, "I ended up going back to school."

First she went to St. Lukes Hospital in Boise for a brush-up course and then to Harborview Medical Center in Seattle for classes. Her travel and housing expenses were partially paid by a private foundation in Boise. She took four weeks of emergency training classes with paramedics, working twelve to fourteen hours a day. She then returned to Boise for more training at St. Alphonsus Hospital.

She was now certified as an "emergency nurse practitioner," and while she handled many trauma cases in a three-room log

[8]Telephone interview, June 17, 1975.

cabin built with donated funds, more and more people began coming to her for primary care. As a protective measure and so she could give better health care to the people near Stanley, Osborn enrolled in the Family Nurse Practitioner Program at the University of Utah.

Along with new training came a new clinic, again built with funds contributed by residents and the many people from all over the country that vacation near Stanley. Dedicated in June 1975, it has two large treatment rooms and a smaller examining room that doubles as a morgue and an X-ray room.

Osborn sees the gamut of medical cases, including – on an emergency basis – some animals, usually the pets of vacationers. "I've seen a couple of goats, a raven, and a cougar with a bad case of diarrhea – really bad," she says. As for the human patients, she sees "everything and anything." This has included heart problems, both angina and coronary, and those stemming from difficulties with the high altitude, accidents with fishhooks, some very bad burns, allergic reactions in all degrees, serious car accidents, drownings, upper respiratory problems (especially when the weather changes), strep throat, Rocky Mountain spotted fever, insulin shock, two stabbings, gunshot wounds, a multitude of motorcycle accidents, and during the past winter some nasty snowmobile accidents. She has also delivered two babies. There are also such problems as colds and flu, plus physical examinations for Forest Service workers and for kids involved in football and other school activities.

Does she consider her nurse practitioner training to have been valuable? "I wouldn't be in this job without it," she said. "My nursing background [she graduated from a four-year program at Ball State in Muncie, Indiana] actually was great but in no way could you take that training and go into this."

Yet the nurse practitioner concept is not a new idea, not even to the Intermountain Region. In the mid-1960s, Dr. Henry Silver helped develop a program as a joint project of the University of Colorado's Pediatrics Department in the School of Medicine and also the School of Nursing. Theirs was a pediatric program in which the nurses, who had to have a master's degree, were extensively trained in most of the duties of the pediatrician. Once accepted, they must spend four months in the University's Medical Center in various nurseries, wards, and clinics. A few of the extensive studies in which they are involved include the complete physical examination, aspects of parent-child relationships, growth patterns, physical and psychosocial development, essentials of infant nutrition, immunization procedures and schedules, personality development, and proficiency in counseling parents in child rearing practices (Silver *et al.*, 1968).

Their first graduate was Susan Stearly, who set up an office and health station in Trinidad, Colorado, the county seat of Las Animas County and core of a depressed coal mining area. Its residents felt the lack of medical care, especially where their children were concerned, since in the 4,800 square miles, there were seven doctors – one for each three thousand residents ("Nurses: Where Doctors Don't Reach," 1966).

Stearly made house calls every morning and in the afternoon held office hours at the health station. Despite the obvious need for her services, at first there were days when no one took advantage of her presence, perhaps because the people were accustomed to managing without help, even when it was needed. Gradually, however, the people recognized Stearly's skills, and within four months she had 45 patients.

Despite the growing number of nonphysician primary care personnel, including the Medex and the nurse practitioner, and the obvious enthusiasm of the many people involved, these programs are not without their problems. The Anderson *et al.* study (1972) found the main difficulties with the concept to be the "limited number of willing preceptors, unclear legal definitions (especially in Montana), and personality conflicts." Disincentives to hire primary care personnel focus on (Anderson *et al.*, 1972):

(1) The physician's legal liability for the primary care person

(2) The limited capacities of the primary care personnel ("another physician would be better")

(3) Their high salary expectations

Idaho, Wyoming, and Utah have enacted legislation concerning physician assistants, which authorizes a specific organization to establish rules and regulations governing their functions and also to approve the physician assistants regarding their education and training qualifications. Montana, however, has only a vague statute which allows the physician to delegate tasks and to supervise a "paramedical specialist" without specifying what tasks. No other law is directed at physician assistants, making it unclear as to whether performing these tasks might institute unlicensed practice of medicine. And no requirements or qualifications for approval of the assistant are specified. There is no regulating agency in Montana.

Since nurse practitioners are licensed and registered to practice nursing, they may of course do so, but only Idaho has enacted legislation specific to the nurse practitioner, making opinions as to a nurse practitioner's role at times foggy.

Personality conflicts can cause problems within any working situation, but when there is a change in role, as with the nurse practitioner, or the creation of a new one, as with physician assistants, professional jealousies may arise. "Nursing has always been its own worst enemy," says Huether. "Nurses need to be educated to understand the role of the nurse practitioner."

Patient acceptance of the new nurses has not been a problem in any way, adds Huether, but physician response varies. "For those who understand that the only thing the nurse practitioner is practicing independently is nursing, acceptance is fine."

National Health Service Corps

The National Health Service Corps marks the first federal effort to provide public health service physicians, dentists, nurses, and other health professionals to areas – urban and rural – where other health resources are inadequate. Established by the Emergency Health Personnel Act of 1970, the Corps is intended not only to meet the immediate "emergency" manpower needs of an area, but also to help communities develop self-sustaining solutions to their local health problems. By July 1975, the Corps planned to have more than eight hundred health professionals, including physicians, dentists, nurse practitioners, and physician assistants, serving in over 250 communities in 46 states.

By law, the Corps program depends upon the participation of many people: The need for health personnel must be certified by the local medical or dental society, the state equivalent society, and the local government for the area concerned. In addition, the state and areawide comprehensive health planning agencies, the regional medical program for the area, independent health practitioners, and consumers must assist in program development. While these requirements may seem cumbersome, they do serve to assure solid community support for health care programs.

To help professionals select the communities best suited to their needs, the Corps conducts an assignee and community selection matching questionnaire. The Corps compiles the information and supplies profiles on communities with requested characteristics. It pays for assignees to make one preassignment visit to the areas of their choice.

The Corps agrees to provide administrative and financial management and assistance. The community agrees to manage the practice and to provide an office, equipment, supplies, and staff support, and it is responsible for purchasing, billing, and collecting fees. Backup services, available through other Corps members, hospital affiliations, and local practitioners, assure assignees that their patients will receive care when they are away for training or vacation. For the few Corps physicians who are in solo practice, a special program of the American Medical Association, Project USA, provides physician coverage for short periods of time.

Corps assignees are salaried members of the public health service, but they charge fees for their services which are returned to the U.S. Treasury. Other financial arrangements – such as prepayment – can be made, and those who cannot pay will not be refused service, but the goal of the fee-for-service requirement is twofold: (1) to emphasize that the Corps is not in an area to undercut existing health providers, and (2) to help build an economic base for an independent, post-Corps medical or dental practice.

In the first two and a half years of Corps operation, 25 percent of its clinic sites have become independent and no longer require direct federal support. While the Corps program is not intended solely for rural consumption, it is mandated by law to place a resident physician in every "doctorless" county of the nation. Most communities with National Health Service Corps personnel have less than one primary care physician for every four thousand people, and 85 percent are located in rural areas.

All 44 National Health Service Corps members in Region VIII (Colorado, Utah, North Dakota, South Dakota, Wyoming, and Montana) are in rural areas, according to Marva Collins,[9] public health adviser to the National Health Service Corps at its Denver office. This includes thirty medical doctors, six dentists, three nurse practitioners, one physician assistant, one child health associate, and three psychiatrists.

---

[9]Telephone interview, March 10, 1975.

With the end of the draft, it might appear that the Corps would have a difficult time recruiting doctors, since a Corps assignment fulfills a military obligation, but there have been no such problems, says Collins. "There are some doctors who want a general practice in a rural community and the Corps helps them get started without their making a big financial investment. Maybe they aren't sure about the practice, maybe they're afraid that this might not be what they want. The Corps gives them two years [the time period for which the Corps personnel commit themselves] with a salary while they are making up their minds."

They can resign at any time, but most stay for two years, says Collins, because of certain advantages. "For example, if the draft would start up again, their military obligation will have been taken care of. Also, they can get loan forgiveness on medical school loans and there is a twelve thousand dollar bonus paid at the beginning of each year, which they have to pay back if they don't finish out the year. A few have stayed in the program longer than two years because they wanted to make a career in the public health service, but most only stay two years."

However, this is not just a two-year program for the town. "It's a continuity of service," says Collins, for after the doctor finishes his or her service period, the National Health Service Corps tries to provide another medical person.

"The National Health Service Corps is pretty much of a bargain for the community," says Collins. "It usually costs them about twenty-two thousand dollars for a doctor, and we've had towns offer us forty-four thousand. They only pay back a percentage of our cost – a percentage of what they collect. This is determined by what our input is and what their input is. Say our investment is twenty-two thousand dollars for the doctor's salary and theirs is twenty-two thousand for equipment, et cetera. Then it was a fifty-fifty investment, and they pay back fifty percent of the money collected in office fees.

"Although the bill passed in 1970, the program didn't get started until 1972. So we really haven't had time to evaluate its success. But we [Region VIII] haven't had any doctors not stay their two years, and we haven't had any towns ask us to remove a doctor."

One Intermountain Area doctor associated with the National Health Service Corps is Mike Barber, 26, a graduate of the University of Indiana Medical School. He practices in Tooele, Utah, but his patients are scattered throughout an area roughly the size of Connecticut, according to the Salt Lake *Tribune* (1974). Barber received a health scholarship while in medical school and, in return, was required to spend two years with the Corps.

"I grew up in Connersville, Indiana – a town the size of Tooele – and have always been interested in rural medicine," he said. "And I have always wanted to practice in a small town. It's great."

One has to learn his or her own capabilities in a rural practice such as his, says Barber. "You just can't refer your patient to another doctor, so you have to be able to take care of it – anything from delivering a baby to setting a broken arm yourself. With the proper training, a rural physician should be able to take care of ninety to ninety-five percent of all the problems he gets."

Transportation is, of course, one of the problems a rural doctor faces, says Barber, for some of his patients must travel fifty miles to see him and probably wouldn't go that far unless they were seriously ill. Another is trauma cases. "You see more traumatic injuries . . . than if you would have a family practice in the city. You get a lot more emergency room patients."

But while recognizing the problems, Barber can also see advantages to a rural practice. "I live with my patients as neighbors and friends. It makes my work easier and makes them closer," he says.

The Rocky Mountain Health Maintenance Organization in Colorado

Mesa County, Colorado, is located in the rural, semi-arid southwestern part of the state. The population is about 55,000, with roughly half of that number living in Grand Junction, the county seat and the business, commercial, and medical center of a 44,000-square-mile section of western Colorado and eastern Utah, an area larger than the entire state of Pennsylvania.

It was here in Grand Junction that one of the first federally assisted health maintenance organizations had its beginning in 1971. The Rocky Mountain Health Maintenance Organization became fully operational as of January 1974 and boasted 74 physicians and an enrollment of more than 7,200 after less than a year of service. A high percentage of those enrolled are on welfare; in fact, one month after a letter detailing the program was sent to Mesa County's 4,600 welfare recipients, four thousand had signed up.

The idea for such a medical organization was conceived by Ward Studt, a local orthopedic surgeon, and Jim Forrester, a local hospital administrator, who took their plan to the U.S. Department of Health, Education, and Welfare's Region VIII offices in Denver and found an encouraging audience. Under the auspices of HEW officials, a meeting was arranged for Grand Junction–Mesa County physicians interested in the development of a health maintenance organization; and after a grant was approved, the Rocky Mountain Health Maintenance Organization was launched. Participating physicians formed into a business-support group to stand at risk for the venture called the Western Colorado Physicians Service Organization.

Rent-free space was immediately found at St. Mary's Hospital, and the Denver-based Colorado–Wyoming Regional Medical Program followed suit by sponsoring a symposium on professional corporations. Fears and hesitancies on the part of the physicians were allayed and participation was stimulated.

As defined by federal law (Public Law 93-222), the Rocky Mountain Health Maintenance Organization in Grand Junction is an independent practice association, or a foundation-type health maintenance organization. As the name implies, a physician may contract as an RMHMO physician and still maintain his traditional private practice. This flexible arrangement seems to work in Grand Junction, substantiated by the fact that each of the 74 RMHMO physicians has an independent, fee-for-service practice in addition to his health maintenance organization commitment.

A Mesa County family (only county residents are eligible), enrolled in the "standard" RMHMO plan at $53.80 per month, can expect full coverage for doctor and hospital bills, laboratory and other preventive and diagnostic tests, emergency and sudden illness care, maternity care (including pre- and post-natal prescription drugs), and care outside Mesa County as prescribed by the RMHMO physician, or in the event emergency treatment is necessary while the member is outside the county. A recent merger with a Catholic Church–affiliated organization, previously known as Community Social Services of Colorado West, will add a broad range of health-related social services to the list of RMHMO benefits.

A single individual can expect the same coverage for $21.80 per month. The monthly premium for a "double" (two members of one family in one household) is $42.80. A "customer" may also choose from the "cost-sharing" plan. The premium for this plan is less, but the coverage is also. Once enrolled, the enrollee is not required to do additional paperwork. For treatment, he or she need only present proper identification.

The Rocky Mountain Health Maintenance Organization is "community rated," meaning that all economic, demographic, and other cost-related factors are taken into account in figuring premium rates. An accepted fee scale, called the "Colorado relative value schedule," dictates the range within which a physician can charge for any given medical service. A peer review committee, made up of elected RMHMO physicians, sees to it that RMHMO physicians' fees fall within the scale, and that all prescriptions and treatments are necessary and justifiable. In fact, individual physicians who affiliate with the organization agree to submit their professional performance to the judgment of their peers.

Victor A. Crumbaker, M.D., medical director of the organization, says that the peer review function is a good quality-control mechanism and describes the process as consisting of keeping a close watch on physician claims and patient records to see that they are reasonable and within the Colorado relative value schedule. In addition, all medical treatments and prescriptions are checked to see that they are reasonable and within the purview of accepted medical standards of practice. "For instance," explains Dr. Crumbaker,[10] "we won't authorize treatment or prescriptions that have no actual therapeutic value."

All physician claims for payment are first screened by the RMHMO accounting office and, if no irregularities are observed, the claim is processed for payment. In the event an irregularity or questionable charge is detected, or when claim is made for a medical procedure or service beyond the capability of the laymen to check routinely, the claim is passed along to the peer review committee.

Has a member physician ever been reprimanded for an overcharge or an irregular practice? "We've talked to a couple of people," replied Crumbaker. "Mostly it's a matter of getting accustomed to the tighter controls. Health maintenance organiza-

[10]Telephone interview.

tion doctors, wherever they practice, will not have the freedom to maneuver that they have in a totally independent practice; and some will always resent the third party influence.

"On the other hand," said Crumbaker, "an HMO affiliation is a real asset to the physician. Most medical doctors are very well trained but not very well educated, and they need help in worldly matters. For instance, I think our own RMHMO is a preferable alternative to dealing individually with the federal government, and this will become especially true for physicians as national health insurance comes on the line. When it comes to matters like that, physicians tend to feel alone and alienated and will appreciate the buffer, the interface that an HMO offers; and, too, our kind of HMO is a moneysaver in that we utilize existing facilities and equipment."

Freedom from worry about bill collecting is yet another advantage of being a member of a health maintained organization, according to Mike Weber, RMHMO comptroller.[11] However, said Weber, doctors risk 20 percent of their fee, which is placed in escrow as insurance against bad debts, overutilization, and other adverse exigencies. If there are no demands on this contingency reserve, the entire amount is returned to the physician, proportionate to his or her earnings.

Reduced paperwork is also a benefit, says Weber, beginning with enrollees who never receive a bill from the doctor or hospital and who never need file a claim form. In fact, individual, standard plan, RMHMO members need not pay their premiums in person, since they are either deducted from the members' paychecks by the employers (because the members are group enrollees) or deducted automatically from their bank accounts (because they are individual enrollees). As for the doctors, druggists, and hospitals – they merely add up their accounts and submit a single bill for a single payment each month.

The system incorporates further paperwork economics by coordinating medical records. A master card file in the RMHMO office for each enrollee contains a summary of pertinent patient information and is updated from physician reports sent in at the end of each day. Even substitute physicians can quickly bring themselves up-to-date by reviewing the patient's card, and be certain that they are not duplicating or contradicting previous

[11]Telephone interview.

treatment and medication. When the volume warrants, the entire system will be computerized and handled automatically.

Local control is another often mentioned "plus" described as being important to RMHMO doctors in light of impending legislation that vests more and more regulatory authority with the state and federal governments. Medical director Crumbaker explains it this way: "To retain local control is a genuine advantage at a time when the shift is to federal controls via such mechanisms as PSROS [public service regulatory ordinances] and national health insurance. The federal government recognizes RMHMO as a vehicle that will let us do just that – govern ourselves, make our own options. Arguments, if any, will be with our own people."

The most popular patient benefits have proved to be the "no limit" on office calls provision and the fact that prescription drugs are paid for, according to Mary Davidson,[12] who is in charge of marketing the plan.

But RMHMO is not without its problems. Davidson says marketing difficulties arise because of misconceptions about the federal role, employer reluctance to keep track of multiple choices, skepticism about the stability of RMHMO, concern over whether a health maintenance organization patient could get care under the plan when he or she is outside the area, and general resistance to change that is found against anything new.

Acceptance of the RMHMO has not been unanimous. About 15 percent of the 95 physicians in Grand Junction–Mesa County have elected not to affiliate with RMHMO. Six general surgeons seem to constitute the hard-core resistance, but all six accept referrals by the organization.

Welfare recipient and RMHMO enrollee, Elzada "Minnie" Dean,[13] previously under the Medicaid program, isn't so pleased with the new arrangement either. "But I'm not sure why," said Minnie, "I guess it's because of my feeling that the doctors aren't as thorough as before – they rush you through – like you're kind of being processed.

"They just treat you routinely. And I don't like having to go to my HMO doctor before I can go to a specialist," she added. "And I think the monitoring they do now is bad because it forces people to leave the hospital before they're really ready, sometimes. Just

[12]Telephone interview.

[13]Personal interview.

because it says on a chart that you're supposed to get well from an operation in five days doesn't mean you're going to.... Actually, I don't see that much difference.... I think it's too soon to tell.... I guess it will all work out, though," was Minnie Dean's thoughtful summary.

Mrs. Rosalie Closser,[14] another welfare enrollee previously under Medicaid, feels substantially more secure with RMHMO. Rosalie, who has the distinction of having only one transplanted kidney donated by her brother three and a half years ago, requires regular and extensive care. She says that "the HMO people are just as nice as they can be. There's no hassle, no red tape, and they always pay my bills on time. That wasn't always true before.... Several times I had trouble getting my bills paid, and they were almost always slow – and with me it's a matter of life or death."

Because of her transplanted kidney, Ms. Closser must take a variety of drugs each day, must have blood tests every two weeks, and must go to Denver for a complete physical examination and for special tests twice each year. She also experienced the need for emergency treatment outside the area, having injured her leg during a visit with relatives in California. "They even paid for all that," said she. "HMO is the answer to my prayers. I don't know what I would do without it."

The Utah Valley Hospital in Provo, Utah

A group practice that is not under a single roof is one way to describe the rural health project based at Utah Valley Hospital in Provo, Utah. Basically, it is a plan where emergency room physicians travel to rural clinics and provide patient care or, when a physician or nurse practitioner is already at the clinic, offer backup and 24-hour consultation services.

Funded by the Robert Wood Johnson Foundation in Princeton, the program has been in operation for sixteen months and hopes are that it will be fully self-sufficient within three years.

The idea for such a plan came to Keith Hooker, M.D., chief of the emergency room at Utah Valley Hospital, after a two and a half year stint as a public health service physician in an Alaskan Eskimo village. In that village, health aides whose only job require-

[14]Personal interview.

ment was that they "be able to understand English and operate a two-way radio," says Hooker,[15] were stationed in outlying areas. Every evening they would radio descriptions of ailments during what public health service doctors referred to as the "agony hour." The physician would make recommendations or, if the situation sounded serious, have the patient flown to the village for treatment.

Back in Utah, Hooker and Dr. Eugene Davie, then emergency room chief at Provo, felt that this same plan (but with the doctors flying to the patients) could be used to provide health care to Utah's isolated rural areas. Hooker's partner was later killed in an airplane crash, and the other physicians (there are now a total of five) prefer to drive, leaving Hooker as the only airborne doctor.

To start a clinic in an area where a physician shortage is felt, personal visits are made to help gain local support. A town meeting is then held to assure public awareness of the plan and to discuss advantages of the program and financing, and allow time for a question and answer session. At this meeting, slides are shown of a typical clinic and a typical clinic day. Economic factors and other facets pertaining to the community's health care, such as distances to nearest facilities, are discussed.

Once the decision is made to establish a clinic, the community must provide the building (which is leased by the hospital for a dollar a year), and the staff and equipment are provided by the group.

Currently, there are clinics in Green River, East Carbon, Fillmore, and Castledale (Utah). All but Fillmore has a nurse practitioner on duty 24 hours a day. Doctors provide at least two clinic days per week, and someone is always at the Utah Valley emergency room for the nurse practitioner to refer to. Communication between clinic and hospital is currently being done by telephone and mail, but Hooker sees computers and other telecommunications systems as the method of the future. Tests can be started at the local clinic and continued at Utah Valley Hospital, if necessary. Pharmacy needs can be supplied by visits from the physician, or the nurse practitioner can call in the prescription to the doctor, who will then call it in to the local pharmacy. Of that practice, Hooker says, "It's cumbersome, but it's legal."

And, an agreement with Four Corners Mental Health Service helps provide health care to the total person.

---

[15]Telephone interview, May 20, 1975, and speech, May 21, 1975.

The rural clinics, which are officially outpatient clinics of Utah Valley Hospital, have the full support of all the hospital staff, including the administrative personnel. Billing and similar paperwork are taken care of by the hospital. Says Hooker, "I can go out and practice medicine and have all that other stuff done for me."

The ultimate idea is that the community can attract a full-time physician, with backup being provided by the Utah Valley Hospital doctors, a nurse practitioner, or both. This plan has recently become a reality in Castledale, where a full-time physician has replaced the three days a week (when a doctor was available) provided by the group. He will have a busy practice, says Hooker, since a normal patient load is four hundred per month; but in Castledale the norm is closer to 850 patients. Utah Valley Hospital physicians provide backup for vacations and perhaps take over one day each week for the new physician.

The situation in Fillmore is somewhat different from the other three in that Utah Valley Hospital provides administrative services only. The community made a contract with the group to take care of the billing and other paperwork, and medical services will be provided by two National Health Service Corps physicians. A nurse practitioner was involved with Fillmore's health care until recently when he quit to work in Salt Lake City.

East Carbon's clinic is run by the United Mine Workers — with Utah Valley Hospital physician services contracted for — and has a full-time nurse practitioner. Two physicians split 51 hours of coverage each week. Green River (population about a thousand) can receive medical care 24 hours a day from a nurse practitioner and two days a week from Utah Valley Hospital physicians. "The population is so small there that the community will never break even on their plan," says Hooker, explaining that all communities have to reimburse the hospital when the clinic doesn't break even. "But that town is exceptional in that the people there pay their bills almost compulsively."

Patients pay $7.00 an office visit, whether they see the nurse practitioner or the doctor, but the Utah Valley Hospital physicians involved are strictly on a salary as far as their rural clinic work goes, says Hooker, and the men are paid $150 per day plus an amount for travel. And while this mode of payment might not always be the best, Hooker said he felt those on a fee-for-service plan would "only be human" and try to see how much they could earn. "In Alaska I got tired of working hard and seeing the guy next to me slough off and get paid the same, but here it's worked out well and the doctors enjoy the private practice. I think it's unique here. I was picky when I hired the two new guys who came in with us – I hired guys who were good GPs and not just in it for the money."

And if $150 a day sounds like a lot of money, it is tempered by the realization that Hooker made $14,000 last year on visits to clinics and had $10,000 in plane expenses. The emergency room work, where the physicians are on duty for 24 hours and then off several days is the "carrot," says Hooker, and the rural health work is the "stick."

Several other towns are interested in getting medical care from Utah Valley Hospital, including one that wants seven days a week, 24-hour coverage and another hoping to receive emergency care from the traveling physicians.

"Things are really changing," Hooker says. "I never know what the situation is like until I come in here each day and talk with the rural health administrator."

But one thing he feels certain is that this is a "unique Rx"; a plan not dependent on any one doctor and that allows a choice of both residence and place of practice to the physician and his family.

Automated Devices in Missouri

Because of a cooperative effort of the University of Missouri School of Medicine and the College of Engineering in Columbia, three rural towns in central Missouri are reaping the advantages of "computerized medicine." Their system is not a full-fledged mode of comprehensive health care delivery; but it is a way of testing the capacity of automated devices.

Originally set up in Salem, Missouri, and funded by the Missouri Regional Medical Program, it was designed to see just how well patients, physicians, and staff could accept automated help. Within the Salem clinic, the computer made it possible for a patient to undergo a full battery of tests in less than three hours, and could compile and bank data in an orderly, retrievable form. Included in the computer's files were sight, hearing, blood pressure, electrocardiogram, blood chemistry, urinalysis, and X-ray results, as well as answers taken in an automated patient history acquisition routine. The physical examination could also be entered when completed by the physician.

It was found to be completely acceptable to all working with it. However, financial difficulties forced the Missouri Regional Medical Program to drop the program and also for the medical school to cut back on the Salem program, but a second grant enabled the beginning of another phase of the project.

Currently, physicians in three Missouri towns are hooked by a special telephone line to a PD-11 computer in Columbia: four family practitioners in Lebanan, a town of about 8,220 population; a solo family practitioner in Mexico, population 12,839; and a group of physicians, mostly specialists, in Moberly, population 13,170. The towns are twelve, 47, and 39 miles away respectively from the medical center in Columbia. One of the areas can, by teletype device, have access to an IBM 360 computer for additional programs.

These computers are currently involved mostly with patient and physician education, says William Allen, M.D.[16] an associate professor at the medical school's Department of Community Health and Medical Practice. Programs such as those on allergies, obesity, hypertension, and diabetes have been entered into the computer. After office personnel show the patient how the cathode ray system works, the computer asks questions and provides visual information on a screen similar to a television screen.

Physicians are provided information by keying in the right code for a certain subject; information is printed on the screen, or a printout can be obtained. The computer is used for diagnosis assistance and also for drug interaction, enabling the doctor to easily find out if a patient on one medication will adversely or positively react to another, or if certain drugs will affect laboratory procedures. Work is also done with the billing process and scheduling.

In the future, the medical school hopes to move ahead with more physician and patient education and also record work. "For example," says Allen, "a physician may see a patient with hypertension and write down only a few words on the record. The doctor by using these 'cue' words can input to the computer and receive a more detailed account for his record." Developing detailed rec-

---

[16]Telephone interview, May 20, 1975.

ords from the "cueing" system, says Allen, is in the experimental stage and is currently a long way from being in common use.

"Our program is really an attempt to see how technology could be helpful to the practicing physician," says Allen. "We wanted to know if a physician could be as close to the medical center as his telephone. And patient time is valuable – we wanted to know if their waiting time could be put to good use. And, could physicians get reference material without going to a library? In many communities it is difficult to acquire the kind of library we have at the medical center, and we wanted to know if the material could be obtained by a computer. However," he added, "financial problems have forced a cutback on experimentation, and only those items that the medical school feels are important are being computerized."

The computer project has been funded by a Department of Health, Education, and Welfare project grant that ran out on July 1, 1975. "We have made an application for another project grant and are looking for other forms of funding, but we really don't know what will happen," says Allen.

Beaufort–Jasper Comprehensive Health Services, Inc., in South Carolina[17]

The health problems in Beaufort and Jasper counties in South Carolina were well documented in the 1960s. Malnutrition, parasite infestation (73 percent of the black children were infested with ascaris or trichuris trichuria), anemia (26 percent of the children), and a lack of health professionals (physicians per thousand population in 1971 was 0.59, and dentists per thousand population, 0.14) were grave problems. Of 25,000 people who met Office of Economic Opportunity poverty guidelines, 62 percent were low-income, were without health insurance, had dilapidated housing, and lacked plumbing facilities or potable water; 58 percent of the black people had an educational level below the eighth grade, and large numbers of unemployed people could not pay for health care or environmental improvements.

To rectify this situation, Beaufort–Jasper Comprehensive Health Services, Inc., was created in June 1970 as a private, non-

---

[17]Material in this section is taken from unpublished material of Beaufort–Jasper Comprehensive Health Services, Inc., Ridgeland, South Carolina.

profit corporation by an Office of Economic Opportunity grant of $754,373. After nine months of planning, staffing, organizing, and setting up facilities, the project leaders opened a main office in the city of Beaufort and four satellite health centers. These are located in Sheldon and on St. Helena Island in Beaufort County and in Hardeville and Grays in Jasper County. A new central facility opened in January 1973 in Chelsea.

The target area of the service is the 22,500 low-income people of Beaufort and Jasper counties. As of April 30, 1974, 5,885 families and 19,578 individuals were registered in the program, which covers thirteen hundred square miles. Beaufort–Jasper Comprehensive Health Services, Inc., has attempted to develop a nine-pronged approach to address the health and development needs of the poor in this two-county area. They are: clinical care; environmental health care; patient health, education, and action; housing; water and waste sewage; land drainage; manpower development; youth programs; and efforts to address the health care and environmental needs of the poor.

The health services project started out with a comprehensive medical team working in and out of each center: a doctor, one or two registered nurses, a licensed practical nurse, three to eight family health workers, a medical records clerk, and a receptionist. Two Medex who had served twenty years as military corpsmen served on two of the teams. The project hired a dentist who works out of a mobile dental unit in Jasper County, which has only one dentist. The area's Head Start Program donated $10,000 toward this unit in return for dental care for children enrolled in the program.

Laboratory facilities for the entire project are set up in one center, and another center has a well-stocked pharmacy. The facilities, loaned or leased from the county's Public Health Department, are well-equipped clinics with examining and treatment rooms, small labs, and interviewing and waiting rooms. Mobile units or trailers alongside each center serve as administrative and records-keeping offices.

The project's services are free to persons whose income is below the poverty guidelines ($3,200 for a rural family of four). Physical examination, treatment, medication, and prescriptions are provided for many rural poor who never before had access to such comprehensive health care.

The short-range objectives of the program are to make a measurable positive impact clinically and environmentally by developing a health care system which includes medical, dental, laboratory, nursing, pharmacy, X-ray, mental health, physical therapy, nutrition, environmental health, health education, social services, and transportation. The long-range objectives are to raise the economic level of the population through manpower and economic development and to provide adequate housing, water, and sanitation. Criteria to measure programmatic success are:

(1) To increase the number of low-income patients treated
(2) To improve the accessibility of health care to the rural poor by having satellite centers and transportation
(3) To reduce the morbidity and mortality of chronic illnesses by early detection, treatment, and health education
(4) To reduce in-patient hospital days
(5) To decrease health problems by improving the patients' physical environment (adequate housing, safe water, and adequate sanitary facilities)
(6) To increase the number of people who are economically self-supporting

The future support of this agency will depend upon the ability of the free enterprise system to supply adequate jobs and income so that the registrants can pay for their own health care. If this does not happen, the agency will continue to depend upon federal funds for support of the clinical care aspects of the program at minimum.

Frontier Nursing Service, Inc., in Kentucky

Established in 1925, the Frontier Nursing Service, Inc., is a plan to help provide medical care to rural Kentucky, using nurses rather than doctors as the nucleus of the services provided. Frontier Nursing Service, Inc., reaches out into the community, with care provided in residential clinics within the community, placing the nurses in intimate contact with their area and its problems.

Mary Breckinridge, its founder and director until her death in 1964, decided to devote her life to the health care of children in rural areas after her own two children died (Frontier Nursing

Service, Inc., 1973). She received her basic training at St. Luke's Hospital in New York and studied nurse midwifery at the British Hospital for Mothers and Babies in London. A member of a prominent Kentucky family, she chose the Kentucky mountains for her project because she believed that, if her plan could be carried out in such an unaccessible place, it could be carried out anywhere.

The base of Frontier Nursing Service, Inc., is located in Hyden, Kentucky (population about eight hundred) and the county seat of Leslie County (population twelve thousand). Approximately 87 percent of the land is mountainous forest, with only 2.5 percent used for farming. The main source of income is logging, followed by farming. Average per capita income is $1,000 a year; about 80 percent of the residents are medically indigent by state standards. According to the publication, "Frontier Nursing Service, Inc." (1973), the land is "tired and eroded, communications inadequate, and roads poor, particularly along the rocky creeks where many of the older people still live."

The nursing service provides primary care for those who live within the confines of its jurisdiction. The care includes (Frontier Nursing Service, Inc., Autumn 1973, Winter 1974):

> ...home health, nursing and hospital clinics, in-patient services, and operates a full-time training program in family nursing and midwifery (nationally accredited) for a total of 22 students with a staff of 65 professionals (five physicians, fifty nurses, one pharmacist, three lab technicians, two X-ray technicians, two research assistants, one social service secretary, and one hospital administrator).... [In 1973] care was provided to a 15,000 population base that included 66,000 ambulatory patient encounters (home and clinic) and 7,000 in-patient care days for 1,750 patients. The service and training [were] provided at a cost slightly below $100 per capita per annum.

In 1973 there were seven outpost centers and a hospital in Hyden, serving a thousand-square-mile area. The outposts have at least two nurses, where initially most of the work uses nurse-midwife skills. Ten years ago, Leslie County had the highest birthrate in the nation – 41 per thousand population – but because of intensive counseling by the nursing service nurses and the increased use of contraceptives, the birthrate has decreased to 18 per thousand population. Family nursing has been stressed recently (a family nurse practitioner program was instituted there in 1969, along with the long-established midwifery school), and it is found that a considerable amount of time is spent with the illness of growing children and elderly people. However, family care has always been a function of the Frontier Nursing Service nurse.

Each district nurse serves from two hundred to 250 families and is responsible for their health. Most of the ailments treated are common respiratory and urinary problems and cuts and bruises. Serious complaints and complicated illnesses are tentatively diagnosed and referred to a physician. Approximately a fourth of the contacts are referred.

A key function of the district nurse is to keep her families well through a broad public health program including innoculations, worm treatments, and instructions regarding sanitary privies, a pure water supply system, child care, and diet.

Until about ten years ago horses were the nurses' mode of transportation, but now rugged jeeps make their way up the creek beds, which is the only way many of the families can be reached. Many of the districts are no more than five miles in radius because the terrain is so inaccessible. No family is more than an hour's travel by jeep, and no outpost is more than an hour from the Frontier Nursing Service's hospital in Hyden, the Mary Breckinridge Hospital.

The Mary Breckinridge Hospital, which replaces the 25-bed Hyden Hospital, has forty in-patient beds, an out-patient department, emergency suite, surgical suite, X ray, laboratory, physical therapy, labor and delivery suite, nursery, library, cafeteria, offices, and classrooms.

The center has more extensive diagnostic and treatment facilities than the nursing outposts, with a resident physician available at all times. It is a receiving center for patients requiring more extensive diagnostic and treatment services, a referral station for specialty care, a consultation center for nurses, and a drug control and dispensing center for the outposts. It is the training center for the Frontier School of Midwifery and Family Nursing and also a research base for university faculty interested in rural problems.

The old Hyden Clinic, according to Isaacs (1972):

> . . . had 23,120 patient visits during the fiscal year 1971 and the outposts had 30,371, making a total of 53,491 outpatient contacts for a population group of approximately 20,000.

In addition, the Frontier Nursing Service cared for 1,902 patients on an inpatient basis, with an average of 3.1 patient days. Simultaneously, the clinic developed and conducted a full-time training program for fourteen family nurse students. These services were performed on an annual budget of $750,000. The staff consisted of four physicians, 41 nurses and nurse-midwives, nineteen aides and licensed practical nurses, one X-ray and laboratory technician, one pharmacist, one social worker, 36 clerical assistants, 63 domestic and maintenance personnel, and a continuous staff of volunteers – young college women, referred to as couriers.

A vast network of consultation, referral, transportation, and teaching services helped supplement the primary health care. Specialty services are available through regional hospitals, university medical centers, regional community health services and other state facilities. Frontier Nursing Service transports many of the patients, and ambulance services are available. Specialty clinics are also conducted on a regular or invitational basis. For example, an orthopedist from the University of Kentucky conducts monthly clinics and a surgical team from the University of Cincinnati conducts biannual ear, nose, and throat clinics. Last year they performed over 50 tonsilectomies for children with recurrent infections. The majority came from medically indigent families, few of whom would have gone to outlying facilities.

This system makes it possible to provide sophisticated health services to the most isolated families without prohibitive costs. Most patients requiring specialty services can be transported to outlying areas at minimum cost. This eliminates the need for rarely used costly equipment and for maintaining full-time specialists.

Some five thousand Kentucky mountain children and their families (more than twelve thousand persons) receive direct and intensive care annually, according to "Frontier Nursing Service, Inc." (1973). In April 1973, at the end of the 48th fiscal year, the Frontier Nursing Service had delivered 16,849 registered maternity cases.

At the end of its first ten thousand deliveries (1925–55) the nursing service has a puerperal death rate of 9.1 per ten thousand live births. Among white women in the United States in this same period, the puerperal mortality rate averaged 34.0 per ten thousand live births.

Says the "Frontier Nursing Service, Inc." (1973):

> The Frontier Nursing Service has had one maternal death in 1,803 live births, or a maternal mortality rate of 1.2 per 10,000 live births between 1950 and 1970. In the state, maternal mortality rates declined from 8 to 2.1 per 10,000 live births during this period. There has not been a maternal death at the Frontier Nursing Service since 1952; and except for 1963 when the county had a flu epidemic, neonatal deaths and still births have declined steadily. (Stillbirths fell from 16.5 to 10.1 per 1,000 live births between 1950 and 1970.)

Over the years Frontier Nursing Service, Inc., has provided hospital care for some 35,000 people and given nearly three hundred thousand immunizations.

The Multicounty Approach in Pennsylvania

During 1967–69, the Pennsylvania Department of Health sponsored a project called "A Demonstration in the Organization of Community Health Resources." The project was funded by the U.S. Department of Health, Education, and Welfare's Health Services and Mental Health Administration. Chosen for the demonstration were five rural counties in central Pennsylvania – Montour, Columbia, Northumberland, Snyder, and Union. The project had three purposes:

(1) To develop local community organizations in the rural areas that would identify and coordinate existing community health services and that would plan and implement supplemental programs
(2) To demonstrate that through committee participation, community leaders would become familiar with and interested in health needs, methods of obtaining financial support, and procedures for implementing program plans
(3) To test a demonstration system for the delivery of health services to rural areas based on self-supportive community action

Through committee organization, local problems were identified, priorities were set, and the most feasible methods of obtaining financial support were determined.

A survey of a thousand representative households was conducted to determine how rural people felt about their own health needs and problems. Task forces were established under local leadership to evaluate identified problems, such as the need to improve emergency health services, the need to coordinate and expand home health services, and the need to provide comprehensive dental care to all children in the area.

In July 1970, the Central Pennsylvania Health Council was established as an outgrowth of the demonstration project, with the project area being expanded to cover eleven counties, for a total population of 575,000. The Appalachian Regional Commission funded the Council (for fiscal 1971) to work with communities in planning a regionwide primary health care delivery system, integrating existing services, projecting new facilities, locating additional resources and coordinating local, state, and federal government involvement.

To date, this cooperative effort has resulted in the establishment of eight primary health care centers, with three more in the planning stage. About 85 percent of the area's 581,000 people will be within less than half an hour's drive from one of these centers, according to Douglas Farber,[18] associate director of development for the Council. There are also a number of related systems that provide links and tie-ins in the overall system: four home health centers, two sheltered workshops for the handicapped and the mentally retarded, two day-care centers, one information and referral service and one of the few vocational-technical high school programs in the country that offers training for dental assistants at the high school level.

For the first three years, the Central Pennsylvania Health Council acts as the organizations' advocate; after that each is on its own and may turn to the Council for technical assistance, but not in a subordinate relationship.

According to the Council's "1974–75 Health Development Plan" (Central Pennsylvania Health Council, December 11, 1974):

> The Central Pennsylvania Demonstration Health Project is firmly grounded on the concepts of self-help, local self-determination, and mutual cooperation. Each project sponsored by the CPHC has, and should continue to have, its own governing entity, usually in the form of a private nonprofit

[18]Telephone interview, May 12, 1975.

> corporation. The board of directors of each institution shall be responsible for all matter pertaining to the planning, development, and operation of [its] projects. The CPHC itself shall at no time enter into the direct provision of patient services. Our concern, instead, is with the development of a viable system of providing the needed patient services with only initial financial support and technical assistance through the CPHC. The basic elements of this system are the independent hospital and community based primary health centers. The centers are the patient's first point of entry into the health delivery system. While these centers must be independently administered in order to remain most responsive to the specific desires of their respective sponsoring communities, they must also cooperate among themselves, and with the neighboring hospitals and other health institutions, to insure the highest quality of patient care at the least possible cost. The greatest emphasis of the CPHC Demonstration Health Project, to date, has been on the development of the individual health centers as sites for the provision of primary health care. This plan proposes that CPHC sponsor additional projects while directing its staff to work intensively toward the development of more and stronger "linkages" both among the centers themselves and with other institutions offering complementary services.

All but one of the primary health care centers are community based and have their own board of directors and an organization established specifically to operate the health center.

Mountain Top Area Medical Center is an example of one of these. Located in Snow Shoe in Centre County, it was the result of the efforts of the local Lions Club. In the late 1960s the members realized that their only physician was nearing retirement age, and they knew it would be difficult to find another doctor who would work fifteen hours a day to care for a hundred thousand people spread across three counties. After exploring options, they contacted the Central Pennsylvania Health Council for assistance and, working with them, secured a grant from the Appalachian Regional Commission, erected a facility, hired medical and dental personnel, and began operation in February 1972. It has expanded its service to include counseling services, home health services, family planning, and health education. According to a Council tabloid (no date), "Few of the 8,000 residents in the Snow Shoe area of Centre County have not benefited from the greatly improved level of health services in the area."

Divine Providence Community Health Service is the lone CPHC hospital-based mode of primary health care delivery. Located in Divine Providence Hospital in Williamsport, it began in late 1972 and offers physicians' services, psychological counseling and referral service, programs in nutrition, and education for prevention of health problems. Emphasis in the program centers on a health team approach. Because close coordination is maintained between various components of the project, the patient is assured a full range of health services.

The CPHC staff is currently concentrating its efforts on strengthening the operating health centers through evaluation, and requested technical assistance, concerning such matters as clinic management, fund raising, public relations work, and so forth.

The Council is also striving to assist the newly formed self-help organization, the Pennsylvania Primary Health Care Administrators Association, Inc., which will serve as a source of pooled administrative services from which the health centers can draw. The Council will assist this organization until it can obtain its own staff; but after it becomes fully operational, CPHC will be able to limit its activity to planning and will not have to become involved in the daily administration of the health care centers.

Also, CPHC will stress development of new primary health centers in areas of critical need, development and strengthening of linkages in the system, and obtaining additional funding for the project. So far, the predominant source of funding has been the Appalachian Regional Commission in cooperation with the Bureau of Appalachian Development of the Pennsylvania Department of Commerce.

Outreach in Kansas

The University of Kansas Medical School has started a program that it thinks brings more doctors to the state's rural areas.

"During the last couple of years we have been working on the premise that an individual is more apt to settle in an area where he took up his last residency," says Charles Brennan,[19] assistant vice chancellor for Health Affairs. "There are statistics to back this

[19]Telephone interview, January 30, 1975.

up. In 1971, Yett and Sloan did a survey – it showed that if an individual gets his M.D. and does his residency in the same state, the probability of staying is seventy-two percent, and if he was also born in the state it is eighty-six percent. For an out-of-state student who gets his M.D. and does not have residency in the state, the percentage is two.

"We've taken that thought and expanded it. We decided to take the opportunity while the resident is here and get him out in the rural areas into a quality program in the state, let him see what's out there, and show him that he won't be isolated from his professional peers. Many fear that they cannot handle this type of practice, and our program shows them that they can."

Called "Outreach," this plan is now three years old. Through it, residents spend two or three months in the rural areas, and are associated with an established M.D. who does the teaching and comes into the university once a month to give lectures and to update his or her knowledge. But, says Brennan, the resident is not just there to look on. "The residents get a good educational experience – an opportunity to see a wider variety of medicine practiced outside the institutions and not just tertiary care. They get an opportunity to do something, to make decisions – they are not just one of twelve trying to put a hand in the wound at the same time. They are right on the spot and have responsibility. It's a total experience – the doctor, his or her spouse, and the family all go. Spouses usually won't tell them where to practice, but they will tell them where not to."

The first Outreach resident went to Garden City, Kansas, a community of about fifteen thousand people. Topeka started with a surgical, then pediatric, and later two medical residents, and then residents were sent to Kingman and Norton.

"We've already reaped some of the benefits of the program, as one or two of the surgical residents are going to return to the towns of their residency to practice," Brennan said. Since "day one" of the medical school, said Brennan, 34 percent of the university's graduated doctors stay in Kansas. "We are now doing a study to see what the retention rate is for students who do their residencies here and not just get their M.D.

"We've been accused of taking students only from the metropolitan areas," said Brennan, discussing the belief that students from rural areas are more apt to return to the country to set up practice. "But in December we finished a study that showed we take more people from rural western Kansas, and they leave just as much as the others do.

"We have some counties where there is no physician at all, and some where the [patient-physician] ratio is five to one. And in many the physicians are alarmingly old. We're trying to fight off a crisis, and we know it will get worse before it gets better. We've increased the beginning class size in an attempt to help – this year's class will have two hundred students; in 1970 it was a hundred and twenty-five. Also, in 1971, we went to a three-year program. We are trying to increase the number of physicians we produce and then retain more through a better residency.

"This problem [doctor shortage] gets put on us – the medical school – and it's not just up to us. We've gone out into the communities and tried to generate interest; sometimes it is difficult to get the physicians to respond as they don't want to give up the time. Then we have trouble in the towns with community pride. Right now, for example, we are thinking of doing a study of Kansas trade centers, to see where they are, and then try to place physicians accordingly. But it's like it was with the consolidated schools; when they started people were upset to find that they might not have a school in their town."

The Presbyterian Medical Services in New Mexico

The Presbyterian Medical Services originated as a branch of the Board of National Missions of the Presbyterian Church, operating the Mission Health Services in the Southwest (primarily New Mexico and Colorado). In 1969, The Presbyterian Medical Services was formed as a separate nonprofit corporation, with an informal relationship to the Presbyterian church.

Service centers are located in the mountain area north of Santa Fe, in north central New Mexico, and across the border in Colorado. The total target area population numbers approximately a hundred thousand, including a large proportion of minorities (Hispanic and American Indian). This population has traditionally faced a number of significant barriers to health care, including low income, lack of health care resources, lack of insight on the part of the consumer as to proper access to and use of the health care delivery system, and geographic barriers.

The overriding purpose of the Presbyterian Medical Services operation is to establish pilot health agencies that will help regenerate communities, delegate operating responsibility and authority as they become possible, and then withdraw as soon as the community can reasonably provide its own health services. The system sees the health care delivery problem as primarily one of poor distribution of physicians and services, and projects a dispersed group of salaried physicians – backed up by specialty services and linked by communications and transportation support – as a mechanism to provide the needed redistribution among scattered rural communities. This concept of group practice relieves some physician distribution problems by providing adequate income and some free time.

A major component of the system is a clinic in Cuba, New Mexico, with ten holding beds, which was funded as a research and demonstration project in 1972 by the U.S. Department of Health, Education, and Welfare. There are five satellite clinics connected with Cuba; and, altogether, about ten thousand people are cared for by the system. It relies heavily on the use of allied health professionals. The 34-bed Holy Cross Hospital in Taos, New Mexico, and an outpatient clinic in Embudo, New Mexico, are a second component of the system. They serve approximately fifteen thousand residents.

With the help of a Robert Wood Johnson Emergency Medical Services Grant, the Presbyterian Medical Services is developing an emergency medical system in a seven-county area of northern New Mexico, in conjunction with the state emergency medical service. At this writing, they are one year into the project.

There are also many "bits and pieces" of medical service that the Presbyterian Medical Services is involved with, according to Robert Clements,[20] vice president of the organization. These include a school health contract with schools in north central New Mexico and the PMS pharmacy, which has a contract with clinical people to supply prepackaged pharmaceuticals for the system and for other medical services.

[20]Telephone interview, May 13, 1975.

July 1, 1975, a grant by HEW for the Sangre de Cristo Health System was awarded to the system. This health delivery system serves approximately ten thousand people through a program oriented toward ambulatory and preventive care, and involves three home health care teams and three diagnostic and treatment centers in Questa (New Mexico) and San Luis and Antonito (Colorado). Contractual arrangements are being pursued with the San Luis Valley health maintenance organization for selected prepaid capitation services to low-income people, said Clements.

The Presbyterian Medical Services group in 1975 consisted of seven physicians and three dentists who provide health care at most system facilities. Services include out-patient and, in the hospitals, in-patient medical care, pediatric care, obstetrics, and a limited amount of surgery. Two ophthalmologists (not system staff) provide services at the clinics several times a month. X ray, clinical laboratory services, and EKG are available. Most centers provide 24-hour coverage.

Consumer boards have been established at each of the system's facilities and are becoming increasingly involved in decisions pertaining to local hospitals and clinics. Consumer boards are also being established in each of the communities in the target area to advise the Presbyterian Medical Services on future development and involve residents in existing programs. Reaction of consumers toward this kind of participation has been encouraging.

Some specialists who are not group members voluntarily provide backup and clinic services. Supporting staff includes laboratory and X-ray technicians, medical records librarians, pharmacists, dietitians, nurses, and clerical workers, most of them employed in the system's hospital and clinics. Salaries in both physician and nonphysician posts are comparable with those paid elsewhere in the area.

The system faces problems common to rural areas: transportation, staff turnover, and the lack of specialty services. The group practice arrangement offers advantages such as salary assurance, relief, backup, referral, ancillary staff, equipment and supplies, and administrative and accounting services, which make remote rural practice more attractive. And the system is exploring alternatives – such as health maintenance feasibility – which would relieve some problems still faced by its staff.

The Rural Extension Clinic in Kirksville, Missouri[21]

The Kirksville College of Osteopathic Medicine in Kirksville, Missouri, operates eleven student-run rural clinics in nearby communities that otherwise would be without medical personnel. In the 1940s six of the sixteen counties surrounding Kirksville had no hospital facilities. Four counties had only small, unaccredited hospitals, and only six counties had registered or approved hospitals.

Of the 104 incorporated cities, towns, and villages in the sixteen counties, only 52 had one or more resident physicians in full-time practice in the community. In addition, there were hundreds of small unincorporated places which served as the primary shopping centers (weekday groceries, gasoline) for extensive farm neighborhoods. Almost without exception, such neighborhoods had no doctors. Ten of the sixteen counties had no county physicians, five had county physicians for the care of county charges only, and in only two counties were there organized county programs aimed at general health education and preventive medical measures. The average population of the towns into which it was hoped to expand rural extension clinics was 273.

Through personal contact with people in the sixteen-county region, it was found that many of the small villages and towns were eager to help establish some sort of health care program. The college people realized that to provide an adequate health service and at the same time to create a training mechanism for their students, the program would have to be established in the communities, not merely by expansion of existing out-patient clinics in the college.

In a study of various methods used by other colleges and communities, a committee found that a common factor seemed to be absent in all programs reviewed: There was no predetermined attempt to prepare the physician by inclination and training for rural practice. The committee felt that actual participation in rural practice while the student was still in school should make him or her much better acquainted with the trials and rewards of a rural practice and, it was hoped, instill a desire to fill this crucial need.

---

[21]The material in this section is taken from that compiled by the Office of Information, Kirksville College of Osteopathic Medicine, Kirksville, Missouri, 1972.

In 1948, Morris Thompson, president of the Kirksville College of Osteopathic Medicine, presented a plan for a rural extension clinic program to the board of trustees of the college. With the board's approval, the program got off the ground in 1949.

Two objectives of the program are primary: (1) to render health services in areas of critical need, and (2) to train the undergraduate osteopathic student in the problems of rural health and the techniques of rural practice, thus interesting him or her in rural practice as a challenging and satisfying life's work. A third objective at the time of the program's inception was secondary but extremely significant at that stage of its development: to gain experience and acquire data which would support the extension and improvement of the program by the college and assist other institutions in the establishment of similar services. Other objectives are: (1) the provision of a demonstration research laboratory in which patients other than indigents serve as teaching material, (2) actual rural practice experience for the future physician, (3) field laboratory for the problem-solving teaching method infrequently used in medical education, and (4) the opportunity for students to develop individual responsibility through community relationships.

A number of factors enter into selection of sites for rural clinics. These factors are urgency of need, number of persons requiring service, interest of people in the community and community health councils, and road systems. The clinics are from nine to sixty miles away from Kirksville.

The actual beginning of the rural clinics program was made in the face of stringently limited funds and personnel. The first clinic was opened in August 1949 in Gibbs, Missouri, a town of approximately 150 people. Through the efforts of the Gibb's Parent-Teacher Association, the clinic was opened in the local post office building. It had a private entrance, a waiting room, and two treatment rooms. The equipment, similar to that supplied for other clinics opened later, consisted of a desk, a heating stove, two leather-topped tables for manipulative therapy, one folding metal army examining table, a metal instrument cabinet, two instrument sterilizers, an army portable operating light, a microscope, and a few minor surgical instruments.

In all cases a town committee or other local organization was responsible for bringing the needs of the community to the attention of the Kirksville College of Osteopathic Medicine and launching campaigns to provide facilities. In 1949, a clinic was opened in Hurdland, at the rear of a general store, in answer to a request by the community. In that year the school board of Green Castle, a town of approximately 350 people, requested and received a clinic. Toward the end of 1949 the Odd Fellows Lodge of the town of Ethel offered to provide a building for a clinic, if one would be established there, and the offer was accepted.

Clinics were subsequently placed in Elmer, South Gifford, Novinger, Downing, Glenwood, Brashear, Baring, LaBelle, Wyaconda, and Bucklin. Clinics in Ethel, Gibbs, and South Gifford were closed in 1970 because of a population shift and reduced need.

Today, equipment and furnishings in the clinics are virtually the same for all. They include adequate waiting room furnishings, treating tables, standard instrument cabinets, floor lights, EKG machines (eight of the clinics have telephone hookups with the Kirksville Osteopathic Hospital for instant professional diagnosis), emergency oxygen units, a centrifuge, a blood analysis unit, microscope, incubator, sterilizer, refrigerator for storing drugs, wooden stools, reception desk and vital office equipment, weight scale, and facilities for minor lab work.

All senior students in the program at the college participate in the Rural Clinic Extension Program for a four-month period during their senior year. Student nurses sent from Northeast Missouri State College occasionally are assigned to work at the clinics. Five supervisors rotate (rotation of supervisors has value in that on different days special problems in different medical facets receive the attention of a specialist).

Students go through an orientation period where they can make a preliminary visit to the chosen community in the company of a senior student who has almost completed service there. This arrangement permits the new student physician to meet future patients on a professional level and helps him or her acquire essential information about the clinic and community.

During the preliminary period, students also receive orientation lectures which provide a working knowledge of procedure and protocol. For example, they learn how to complete death certificates and how best to comfort and deal with relatives of the deceased, and how to handle insurance coverage and claims for themselves and their patients.

Among the student physicians' duties are the following: consultation on individual and family health problems, diagnosis and treatment of specific illnesses, prognosis reports and follow-up observations, and provision of the type of health care the families in their communities might expect from a family physician.

The program has also made it possible for many communities to have fairly comprehensive health programs in their school systems. The students are assigned to specialty clinics, school health examinations, and preventive health programs and immunization clinics upon request of the school. Student physicians lecture on request to local groups and provide a preventive medicine laboratory in the school.

When a student physician is needed after clinic hours (1 to 8 p.m. on Mondays through Fridays and 10 a.m. to 5 p.m. on Saturdays), a call is made to the Kirksville Osteopathic Hospital operator, and the doctor on call is notified. However, the families often become attached to their "own" doctor and prefer his or her care to the doctor on call. In these cases, the desired doctor is contacted.

Numerous home visits enable the student doctor to gain valuable experience in the diagnosis and treatment of illnesses without elaborate technical assistance. If medication is required, student doctors check their opinion with a supervisor and prescribe the necessary drugs. The student physician at all times has full access to facilities of the school clinic and hospital for consultation and cases calling for hospitalization.

Minimal charges are made to help defray operational costs of the rural clinics. A clinic fee of $3.00 ($4.00 in LaBelle and Bucklin to help pay the receptionists' salaries) is charged patients who can afford it, but no patient is denied health care for lack of funds. House call fees are $5.00 and 50 cents for mileage in town and 10 cents per mile for out-of-town calls, but once again, the fee is not imposed on those in dire financial straits. Because the "doctors" offer their expertise a few months prior to receiving their degrees, no professional stipend is awarded them for their services. Medication is available to patients at a standard hospital rate.

Some financial aid was available after 1960 through a Kresge Foundation gift of $20,000 to the college after required matching funds of $60,000 were collected by the school. The current primary financial stumbling block for the program has been its inability to recover costs from Medicare and Medicaid. In 1971, about 32 percent ($62,000) of the billed income of the clinics was written off by the college because reimbursements were not made for health care provided to Medicare and Medicaid patients. The program is trying to obtain certification from the American Osteopathic Association for clinics to be categorized as clinics of Kirksville Osteopathic Hospital. If this goal is reached the U.S. Department of Health, Education, and Welfare will ask the Missouri State Division of Health to inspect the clinics for their certification. When this is done, cost reimbursements for a share of Medicare and Medicaid dollars will be made to the college. One of the methods being considered for creating a situation which will lend itself to certification is a closed circuit television monitor device with a two-way audio system, by which means doctors may audit clinic situations and provide assistance immediately.

All students associated with the rural clinics are required to attend conferences held in the hospital staff room three mornings each week. At these conferences the students and staff members discuss current professional affairs, including problems in administration and public relations, listen to lectures, or present cases. Constructive criticism on a professional level is permitted during case discussions. The students also have meetings which are attended only by the participating clinic personnel.

Individual conferences between the student and his or her supervisor are held in the clinic office to consider specific patient, personnel, and professional problems. This is also where such matters as insurance and hospitalization forms are completed and signed. Hospital procedures are checked for completeness and accuracy, therapeutic procedures reviewed, and financial and other statistical records reviewed and filed.

While working in the clinics, the students are encouraged to take an active part in community affairs, to gain insight into other aspects of a family physicians's life. They spend some time each day in casual visits about the business district of the community, take part in pie suppers, church socials, town meetings, and community improvement programs.

The Rural Health Associates Program in West Central Maine

The Rural Health Associates program in west central Maine is a pilot health care services plan which treats the feasibility of delivering comprehensive preventive, educational, and crisis health services to a rural population through a single delivery system. West central Maine comprises approximately nineteen hundred square miles of timberland, mountains, and farmland. Wood-related industries, such as sawmills and paper factories, are the largest employers among the thirty thousand residents, but the pay is low. The other primary employer is the shoe industry, but production in this and the wood industry has diminished recently, resulting in high unemployment. Agriculture, once a major industry, has all but disappeared. With low income added to the problem of few physicians, health care has been limited, according to Ron McAllister,[22] comptroller for Rural Health Associates.

The program's development began in the spring of 1969 with research into the health needs of the region. With this as background, a staff of the Franklin County Community Action Council began working with local physicians and citizens to secure planning funds for comprehensive health care services. In October 1970, an Office of Economic Opportunity grant made possible the hiring of a small planning staff.

An advisory board was formed to assist the planning staff, which included about 50 percent consumers as well as representatives of health care delivery organizations, business and labor leaders, and other citizens. After reviewing state statutes and regional needs, the group chose a nonprofit health services corporation as the most effective vehicle for bringing the desired programs. Rural Health Associates, incorporated in August 1971, sought and received Office of Economic Opportunity funding for startup. Its program reflects fundamental decisions based upon needs and the organizing group's philosophy (American Medical Association, July 1972):

(1) Health care should be provided through a single system of delivery, a "one door" policy for all consumers.

(2) The system should operate (and physicians be paid) to keep people well. Therefore Rural Health Associates chose to develop a prepayment program. Currently, the prepaid portion is with the federal government. Low-income people who apply to become members are accepted and have comprehensive health care provided by the program, with Rural Health Associates receiving a monthly capitation premium for the family from the

[22]Telephone interview, May 13, 1975.

U.S. Department of Health, Education, and Welfare. Others pay by the fee-for-service plan.

(3) An increase in outpatient services is essential to an overall reduction of health care costs. However, in a rural area it would be both physically and financially harmful for the patients to centralize services exclusively. Thus Rural Health Associates decided to establish ambulatory care centers in outlying areas, as well as an ambulatory center attached to the existing hospital. There are three outlying ambulatory centers: two in Kingfield and Rangely, which are manned by physician assistants who are in turn backed up by regular visits from the central unit's doctors. Both of these units are connected to the central unit by closed circuit television. The third outlying ambulatory unit is in the Jay–Livermore Falls area and is managed by two full-time physicians. All three centers keep regular working week hours.

(4) To enhance the efficiency of the system, allied health personnel will be trained to run the ambulatory centers when physicians are not available and to relieve physicians of routine tasks. The priority placed on preventive health care leads logically to formulation of health teams, training, and using residents and others as allied health personnel and outreach workers.

(5) To maximize and coordinate services to the area, Rural Health Associates will work with other health providers and planners; e.g., the University of Maine, the Franklin area mental health agency, the Androscoggin Home Health Agency, within the region.

The main center, located in Farmington, houses seven physicians, one dentist, a hygienist, and the administrative offices. An optometrist and an ear, nose, and throat physician are also on the staff, and an orthopedist comes in once a month. People needing other specialists are referred elsewhere, says McAllister.

Rural Health Associates stresses health education programs and has held several clinics, including a dietary clinic and a prenatal clinic. Tapes and projectors have been set up in each center so that people can push a button and see demonstrations on such topics as a breast self-examination, high blood pressure, child care, and dental care.

The enrollment of families is a carefully developed part of the program's health education activities. Each family is enrolled personally and carefully informed about the nature of the program, stressing that the center will not be allowed to accept crisis care only and outlining the program's services and the family's responsibilities for health care.

As of the first quarter of 1972, 125 families (more than five hundred individuals) had been enrolled and by June 1975, membership had climbed to roughly fifteen hundred families, or 4,600 people. Families can choose their own physician among the nine on the staff, working out health care plans together. A dental component is also operative, with the dentists stressing preventive care.

Rural Health Associates offers social services through eight "family health workers." These are area residents, trained by the local branch of the University of Maine to do case finding, family registration, and home health education. Transportation is still scarce – the project has two minibuses and provides emergency transportation, but most patients must rely on private cars.

A subsidiary, but essential, goal of Rural Health Associates has been to provide conditions that will attract and hold physicians. To overcome the familiar drawbacks of rural practice, the project plans internal peer review, systematic record keeping, and evaluation aided by the computer, plus required continuing medical education. Physicians rotate duties so that each can spend the necessary time in regular, formal programs. Telecommunication access to specialists, medical centers, and consultants is projected by means of expanding the system already designed.

Rural Health Project, Inc.. in California[23]

Rural Health Project, Inc., demonstrates that a group of private physicians, with the collaboration of the County Medical Society, can responsibly and efficiently conduct a program to provide comprehensive medical care to indigent patients. Rural Health Project, Inc. is an experimental project organizing care for the indigent while offering a base for comprehensive health planning at the local level.

[23]Data in this section are from Rural Health Project, Inc., unpublished material, King City, California, 1974.

The basic objective of the program is to provide comprehensive, high-quality medical care – a "one door" system – to all residents of the area. To this core of single-system health care delivery is attached a variety of services designed to meet the special needs of a large disadvantaged portion of the population. Care is provided in the same facilities and by the same staff for all; only the payment mechanisms vary.

Rural Health Project, Inc., was originally funded by the Office of Economic Opportunity; in 1970 financial responsibility was transferred to the U.S. Department of Health, Education, and Welfare. The Monterey County Medical Society is grantee for the project, and the Southern Monterey County Medical Group (plus a physician in Soledad) is the principal provider of services. This arrangement demonstrates the possibilities for involvement and initiative on the part of local physicians and their professional organization.

The physicians of the Southern Monterey County Medical Group are a private group practice covering general practice, surgery, pediatrics, and radiology. A pediatric nurse practitioner, obstetrics nurse practitioner, and physical therapist also give direct patient care in the group. There is a visiting consultant staff of nine physicians and two psychiatric social workers for specialized services. The group operates a major clinic in King City, with a satellite office in a neighboring town. The George L. Mee Memorial Hospital and Pioneer Hacienda Nursing and Convalescent Home in King City collaborate in the project for in-patient services and extended care. The California State Medical society assists in ongoing service evaluation through peer review.

The target area has two thousand square miles and a population of approximately 22,000, with 3,700 in King City. Nearly 25 percent of the population are below poverty guidelines, and about 40 percent are considered poor. Until recently, approximately six thousand additional needy migrant workers entered the area from March to October, but agricultural mechanization has reduced the flow substantially and the project's principal target is now local residents. Agriculture remains the area's primary source of income.

Physician services at the clinics, and laboratory and X-ray services at the hospital are offered weekdays and in the adjacent hospital emergency room manned by group physicians for nights and weekends. During the summer, clinic evening hours are maintained. The only charges for services to lowest income beneficiaries of the project are a dollar fee (waived on request) per prescription filled and a part of the cost of normal deliveries. A recent "co-pay" program allows low-income community residents above poverty guidelines to receive services on a part-pay basis with the Department of Health, Education, and Welfare grant assuming the balance of the cost. About 8,400 residents of the area are eligible for the program.

Eligible patients receive treatment in the same manner as self-sustaining patients: They make appointments, are given a thorough medical evaluation, and establish a continuing relationship with a physician and other members of the health team. In this manner, not only is treatment for current medical problems provided, but the patient is also taught proper use of routine preventive care. Four station wagons and one small van transport patients from all sections of the project area to the clinics and hospitals when personal transportation is unavailable (American Medical Association, July 1972).

In addition to medical services of physicians, dental service is provided by the project's own clinic. The modern facility contains seven operators and is staffed by two dentists, a hygienist and supportive personnel. Medicines prescribed by local doctors may be obtained at any of the private pharmacies in the target area. Patients with 100 percent coverage pay the first dollar for each prescription with the project paying the balance. Program recipients are provided vision care and appliances. These services are available from a local optometrist, with Medi-Cal rates applying.

A community health services agency is responsible primarily for facilitating delivery of health care to the target population. Community health workers assist eligible families in obtaining medical care by helping them with medical and dental appointments, arranging needed transportation and explaining how and why different forms of medical care are provided. The community health workers have been formally trained to provide information on nutrition, tuberculosis, venereal disease, cancer, family planning, child care, and care of the sick at home.

Public health nurses and social workers are used to provide continuity of care and make families aware of other resources. There is also a health educator-community advocate responsible for disseminating information on health care and health planning and for implementing health education programs.

The Samaritan Health Service in Arizona[24]

Recognizing the problems of rural hospitals, the Samaritan Health Service of Phoenix, Arizona (presently a system of four urban and two rural hospitals with a clinic at the Grand Canyon National Park), took steps in 1968 to bring under its corporate umbrella four rural hospitals with a total of 89 beds: Holbrook Hospital, Navapache Hospital in Lakeside, Grand Canyon Hospital, and White Mountain Communities Hospital.

Since that time, Holbrook Hospital has been returned to the community for various reasons, but all have benefited from the Samaritan plan. Personnel in the outlying hospitals are given refresher courses at Good Samaritan Hospital and special health personnel from the hospital are sent to the outlying hospitals when their services are needed. Resident physicians in the outlying hospitals can confer daily by telephone with experts at Good Samaritan Hospital. Patients with critical and complicated illnesses are flown to Good Samaritan for treatment.

In the opinion of the U.S. Department of Agriculture (July 1973):

> A good part of the consortium's job had been keeping the outlying hospitals supplied with doctors and nurses.... [The] outlying hospitals' access to sophisticated medicine has also been improved. These hospitals can now offer medical tests that are impossible to perform in their small hospital laboratory. A car makes a circuit of each hospital daily and picks up samples to be tested in the Good Samaritan laboratory. The results are telephoned back to the individual hospital. Dieticians from Good Samaritan travel to the smaller hospitals and help them plan their meals. Other experts help set up better billing systems and community relations campaigns — services that small hospitals couldn't afford on their own.

In addition, as a result of the vast improvements in the quality of care provided by these rural hospitals over the last five years, the Joint Commission for Accreditation of Hospitals had given three hospitals accreditation as of June 1974. Grand Canyon is now an out-patient clinic and is unable to be accredited as a hospital.

---

[24] Data are from the Samaritan Health Service, Phoenix, Arizona.

Before joining the Samaritan Health Service, Navapache Hospital, for example, was experiencing the typical problems inherent in rural facilities – financing, understaffing, and lack of physicians. It soon underwent dramatic changes in service capability after the merger, as discussed below.

Nursing. Prior to lease, the hospital provided nursing service. However, the service was understaffed, and it was difficult to recruit nursing staff commensurate with the need. In 1970, Samaritan Health Service provided a cadre of nurses from Good Samaritan Hospital to rotate to Navapache Hospital to provide the needed manpower. In addition, consultation was made available. By 1971, the needed manpower had been recruited. The cadre of nurses from Good Samaritan Hospital ceased at that time.

Anesthesiology. Prior to affiliation with Samaritan Health Service, anesthesia was provided by a local private practice physician on a fee-for-service basis. After the lease was made, a certified registered nurse anesthetist was hired (splitting her time with Holbrook Hospital). In late 1972, a full-time anesthetist was hired for Navapache Hospital.

Electrocardiology. A local practitioner provided this service on a fee-for-service basis prior to 1969. In addition, an outside contract existed with Phoenix cardiologists for phonotraces. After the merger, the affiliation with the local practitioner was dissolved and the outside contract was maintained. The phonotrace was also expanded to include ties with cardiologists at Good Samaritan Hospital.

Diagnostic Radiology. Prior to the lease a private general practitioner provided this service on a fee-for-service basis. This arrangement was terminated subsequent to the merger, and a contract with a group of radiologists from Flagstaff was obtained. A major improvement was the addition of fluoroscopy to this department.

Laboratory – Pathology. A contract with a pathologist in Globe, Arizona, in conjunction with Desert Samaritan Hospital in Phoenix, was and still is the manner in which pathology services are obtained. At present, when special laboratory procedures are needed, a commercial firm is retained.

Pharmacy. A hospital drug room, supervised by the nursing director, provided the only pharmaceutical service before affiliation with Samaritan Health Service in 1969. Since that time, a registered pharmacist has been made available, and the pharmacy has become a separate department of the hospital.

Medical Records. No organized medical records department existed at the hospital before the lease arrangement. After the merger, consultation was provided by the medical records department at Good Samaritan Hospital. In 1971, a full-time hospital medical records director was employed, and the medical records area was designated a separate department.

Food Service. Although this area held the status of a department prior to lease, it was inadequate, and functioned without a dietitian. Following the merger, dietary consultation was engaged from Glendale Samaritan Hospital and Good Samaritan Hospital.

Maintenance. In 1971, maintenance was elevated to department status, and sharing occurred with the central Samaritan Health Service maintenance pool in the care and upkeep of electronic equipment.

The Student Loan Program in Illinois

In 1946 the Illinois State Medical Society and the Illinois Agricultural Association agreed to participate in a program that was designed to provide physicians for rural areas in Illinois. According to Mattson *et al.* (1973):

> ...A fund was established for loans to medical students who would agree to practice in rural areas of the state. The Medical Student Loan Fund Board (MSLFB) with representatives from the two organizations was formed to administer this loan program.... [D]uring a 1948 meeting of the MSLFB, it was decided that the University of Illinois College of Medicine should be asked to set up a program for selecting candidates for admission who intended to serve as rural physicians. It was felt that the need for rural physicians was such that students with the desire to practice in rural areas should be accepted even though their academic credentials were somewhat below those of students normally admitted. Interest in the program was sufficient that a resolution was formally adopted by the 1949 General Assembly of the state to the effect that the Board of Trustees of the university give "definite preference" to applicants from needy areas who at the time of their applications express an intention to return to their home communities upon completion of their medical courses.

> In response to this resolution and the request of the MSLFB, the University of Illinois College of Medicine agreed to receive recommendations from the board for as many as ten students annually. Applicants to the program are usually referred by local farm bureaus, local medical societies, premedical advisers, or former members of the program.... [In] each case the applicant completes the usual formal application to the College of Medicine. On the basis of this application, certain candidates are chosen for interviews with the MSLFB. This initial screening is carried out jointly by officials of the MSLFB and personnel of the Office of Admissions of the Medical Center Campus.

According to Stehr *et al.*, the remaining applicants are interviewed annually by the Student Loan Fund Board. The interview is conducted to evaluate the applicants from the standpoint of suitability and motivation to rural practice; the success or failure of the program is considered to hinge on this critical process. Applicants are interviewed by the entire board which consists of three members of the board of directors of the Illinois Agricultural Association and three rural physicians appointed by the Illinois Medical Society. Representatives of the University of Illinois Admissions Committee are present and may ask questions for their own information, but have no vote. Suitable students are then ranked from highest to lowest, and this list is given to the admissions committee of the University of Illinois College of Medicine, which evaluates scholastic viability. The University of Illinois notifies the committee when acceptances have been made, and simultaneous notice is given to the applicants of acceptance or rejection by both the Medical Student Loan Fund Board and the University of Illinois.

Students receiving recommendations and the rest of the student body are eligible for a loan. The total loan amount per student has varied from $625 per semester to the present amount of $750 per semester, issued at 2 percent interest. At present, students are asked to begin repayment of the principal amount on January 1 of the fifth year following graduation from medical school. Students are asked to pay the interest annually on their notes. During the life of the program, only two students have defaulted on their loan contracts.

Students receiving a recommendation agree to practice for five years in an Illinois town serving a rural area. Students requesting loan assistance are obligated for one year of practice for each year that financial aid is given.

When the program originated, certain Illinois counties were specified as prime areas of need. These areas were reviewed annually and changes were made as new doctors established practices in a county. A population of five thousand or less was the original requirement. During the years, various changes have been made in defining a suitable rural practice location. At present, there is no population figure, and each request is considered individually by the Medical Student Loan Fund Board. All students, including those who have received additional post-graduate training, are asked to establish a family practice in an area of need which serves rural people.

Should students desire to change their plans and not serve in a rural area, they have the opportunity of repaying the total loan amount at 7 percent interest, plus a $5,000 liquidating damage fee. Students receiving a recommendation only from the Medical Student Loan Fund Program may pay $3,000 liquidating damages to be released from the rural practice requirement.

An attempt is made to maintain personal contact with the participants, including an annual dinner meeting held at the medical school for participants and alumni. Students are required to keep the committee informed of their plans for post-graduate education and up-to-date addresses, and must report on their tours of duty in the armed forces.

As for problems with the plan, in recent years more people have been accepted into medical school, and as a result the fund is inadequate to meet the requests for loans. The long payback delay and low interest make the revolving fund somewhat inefficient. Foundation support is being sought to remedy this. Most participants now take residencies and, in addition, serve in the armed forces before establishing practice. This prolonged cultural displacement from a rural setting may result in an increased defection rate. This is hoped to be overcome, somewhat, by giving one half-year credit for each year of post-graduate training in downstate Illinois. This is based on the known correlation between practice location and the site of final post-graduate training.

As of 1972, 266 students had participated in the program. That same year, 24 applicants were accepted by the University of Illinois for medical training through the program.

University of Florida Rural Clinic

In 1969 the University of Florida's College of Medicine (Division of Ambulatory Medicine and Community Programs of the Department of Medicine – now the Department of Community Health and Family Medicine) chose to establish a community-oriented, comprehensive health care service in cooperation with the residents of doctorless Lafayette County.

Located in north central Florida, Lafayette County is about sixty miles from Gainesville and the university there. The Suwanee River is its easternmost border with most of the 2,800 residents living along the river bottomland. The major industry is farming – cattle, dairy and tobacco predominate. There is a small boat building factory in Mayo, and six hundred people work for a pulp mill in an adjacent county, the major source of employment. Median family income is approximately $2,500 to $3,000, and the average educational level is approximately eighth grade. Between three hundred and four hundred black residents live in an area known as "the quarters." There had been no private physician in Lafayette County for ten years.

In Mayo, a recently constructed county health clinic, which housed the office of the county health nurse, offered ample space for the ambulatory care of all residents and became the base of operations for the Lafayette County Health Center. The clinic was designed to serve four purposes:

(1) To provide a teaching and training experience for medical and nursing students and house staff in community medicine. To be effective, this experience would have to be far enough from a medical center to have its own identity, but not so far that it makes traveling burdensome. Students who live and participate in the community could see firsthand how people identify their own needs and how medicine might begin to meet these needs.

(2) To furnish medical services to a community where they had not been readily available.

(3) To establish for the College of Medicine a facility where the problems of getting health care to people and getting people in need of health care to health professionals may be critically studied.

(4) To demonstrate the effectiveness of cooperative participation among all health professionals, patients, and community members.

The Community Advisory Committee, comprised of citizens of Lafayette County, was subsequently reorganized into the Public Health Trust. It was initially formed to help in the planning and operation of the clinic. Because the members of the committee insisted on a fee-for-service plan for those able to pay, the clinic has been self-supporting, which has emphasized that the project is not directed primarily at indigents. Approximately two-thirds of the residents pay for services, thus making the clinic currently almost self-supporting. After three years in operation, it averaged seven thousand to eight thousand visits a year (of 2,800 residents), and had taken over the Lafayette County Health Department responsibilities.

Clinic operations are streamlined to meet community and student needs. One resident in medicine, three or four medical students, senior nurses, and a public health nurse live in Mayo. Personnel from the University are paid a small stipend to cover additional living expenses, and they staff the clinic from 8:30 a.m. to 9:00 p.m. The resident or a faculty member is on call 24 hours a day, seven days a week. About 80 percent of the medical students and 50 percent of nursing students rotate through this clinic experience. In addition to providing care in the clinic or at home, the resident and students write a health column for the local weekly newspaper, and a monthly "Health Letter" is mailed to each residence in the county. The staff participates in the community by assisting science teachers in high school and giving talks to local service clubs and church groups. Faculty members supervise the project on site as often as four days a week.

The Lafayette County Health Center had been so successful in meeting the needs of the community and the medical school that the university extended its efforts into the adjacent doctorless county of Gilchrist. In the county seat of Trenton, the medical school is testing the feasibility of physician assistants delivering primary health care, with part-time physician supervision. Gilchrist County, population 3,550, is located thirty miles west of Gainesville. Agriculture is its major source of revenue, and per capita income is $1,500. Gilchrist County had no physicians, no hospital, and no nursing home. Community efforts to recruit a physician had been fruitless, and in 1970 a local committee approached the Department of Community Health and Family Medicine for help in solving the problem.

Working together, the university and community residents devised a program which would deliver health care to the people and afford a testing model for the medical school. A "local bill" passed by the Florida State Legislature provided startup funds for the purchase of an existing clinic and allocated approximately $10,000 per year for three years to subsidize operations. The bill also created the Gilchrist County Medical Board, consisting of five community members appointed by the governor. County commissioners authorized $5,000 for medical supplies and equipment. Another state bill authorized the employment of physician assistants, and two graduate physician assistants were hired. The medical board was expanded to include nonvoting advisory members from the local health department, the medical school, a correctional institution located in the county, and from outlying communities in the county not otherwise represented.

The clinic is equipped with an X-ray machine and an incubator for office bacteriology. Major laboratory tests are mailed to a clinical laboratory. An electrocardiogram is producing computer-read EKGs through a telephone link. The EKGs are reviewed by the attending physicians. Supervision of clinic activities is provided part time daily by members of the Department of Community Health and Family Medicine, one of whom is available nights and weekends by telephone.

Clinic staff consists of two physician assistants and a receptionist-bookkeeper and a licensed practical nurse, both residents of the county. Both physician assistants and medical students rotate through at various periods. Patients are usually seen by appointment, with nonresidents of the county being seen only in cases of emergency. Office hours are from 9:00 a.m. to 5:00 p.m., with the physician assistants alternating night and weekend emergency calls. The physician assistant takes a history, performs the indicated physical examination and laboratory or X-ray procedures, and either treats the problem or asks the attending physician to see the patient. If the attending physician is not present, but the problem can be solved by telephone, the attending physician is called. Every patient visit is reviewed by the attending physician.

The project's success depends on acceptance – by the community, physicians and physician assistants – of the concept, and on the quality of treatment. The Trenton clinic seems to have gained the support of all three groups. The university plans ongoing evaluation of the system, with eventual addition of studies on quality of health care through computerized medical record data and two-way television and audio equipment, linking the clinic and the university hospital.

Successful results in Lafayette and Gilchrist counties have helped spur the opening of two more rural health projects. Says Dr. Richard C. Reynolds,[25] of the University of Florida College of Medicine:

> Presently we are extending medical services to another county where there are five physicians, supplementing their care through the use of residents in a small 30-bed hospital. Beginning July 1, 1975, we will open another clinic utilizing an amalgam of residents, physician assistants and medical students.

Northwestern United States

In the northwestern part of the United States, there is a group called WAMI, an acronym standing for the states of Washington, Alaska, Montana and Idaho. An experiment in decentralized medical education, its objectives are to increase the number of places in medical school without a major construction effort, increase the number of primary care physicians throughout the WAMI states, improve the health of WAMI residents, expand continuing education programs for health care professionals, broaden education experiences of future doctors by using clinical facilities in various communities, expand the financial base for medical education by encouraging states to pay for the education of their own residents, and assist adjacent states with the development of health professionals' education and correct the maldistribution of physicians in the WAMI region.

There are two phases to the program. The first is the "university" phase during which the students receive their first year of medical education at a school in their home state: the University of Idaho, Washington State University, University of Alaska,

[25]Personal correspondence, March 21, 1975.

Montana State University, or the University of Washington School of Medicine. At the beginning of their second year, all students go to the medical school in Seattle for the remainder of their education. It is hoped that this decreased first-year burden on the medical school will enable it to enroll more students.

The second phase begins at the end of the basic curriculum and is the "community phase." Both medical students and those doing their residency can participate. This phase is spent partially at the University of Washington School of Medicine and partially with physicians in communities throughout the four states. These community medical clinics have been established in areas where it is felt there is the greatest need: family medicine, internal medicine, psychiatry, pediatrics, and obstetrics-gynecology.

Two students or one student and a resident are placed in a community clinic at one time. Student clerkships last six weeks; resident clerkships last six to eight weeks, depending on the time available on the rotation calendar.

The idea for the plan originated in 1969 and by September 1971, nine students began part of their medical education at the University of Alaska. Montana State University became the fifth and final university to enter the program in 1973, and by that time forty students were in the program, equally divided among the four states.

Courses at all universities are equivalent to those taught at the University of Washington School of Medicine. Courses are designed jointly by faculties of all participating universities; performance on common examinations taken by the WAMI students has been indistinguishable from those not involved.

The first two community clinical units were established in family medicine in Omak and Grandview, Washington, in March 1971. Eleven more have been added in Oak Harbor, Anacortes, Spokane and Wenatchee (Washington), Kodiak and Anchorage (Alaska), Treasure Valley (including the cities of Boise, Caldwell, and Nampa) and Pocatello (Idaho), and Great Falls, Missoula, and Billings (Montana). These can accommodate more than 240 students and residents per year, equivalent to the space for 26 full-time students and thirteen full-time residents. It is felt that by having a resident with the student at a clinic, the teaching burden is partially removed from the physician.

Participating physicians are paid for both their work in the community and for their educational effort at the University of Washington, where they come two to four times a year for orientation, education, and planning. Each unit is visited by a "home-based" member of the medical school faculty at least once every six weeks.

Several principles have been learned about this type of education during the WAMI experience. It has been found that a knowledgeable coordinator with curriculum and financial authority must be at each university. Participation of at least eight students at each university is required to develop group cohesiveness; thus students do not feel isolated. One quarter or one semester is the most that any university without experience in medical education should offer during the first and second years of the experiment. In many cases, new courses must be developed. A higher percentage of WAMI students have chosen to go into family practice (62 percent) than those non-WAMI students (47 percent). Of the first 97 students who spent a six-week clerkship in family medicine at the community clinics, 79 (82 percent) are still pursuing careers in family medicine. Limited medical library resources are available at the WAMI areas, therefore making it necessary to develop library resources at each university and community site. Communications between the participants is of utmost importance. To survive, WAMI states will have to assume full financial responsibility for their students (Schwarz, 1974).

Selected References

American Medical Association. *Health Care Delivery in Rural Areas.* Chicago: American Medical Association. July 1972.

Anderson, Craig; *et al.* "New Health Practitioners (NHPS) Market Study." Under direction of Robert L. Kane, M.D. Salt Lake City: University of Utah, College of Medicine. 1972. Unpublished material.

Central Pennsylvania Health Council. "1974–75 Health Development Plan." Lewisburg: Central Pennsylvania Health Council. December 11, 1974.

————. "How Central Pennsylvania Deals with the National Health Care Crisis." Tabloid. Lewisburg: Central Pennsylvania Health Council.

Frontier Nursing Service, Inc. "Frontier Nursing Service, Inc." Hyden, Kentucky, 1973.

______________. *Quarterly Bulletin* (Autumn 1973, Winter 1974), vol. 49, nos. 2 and 3.

Isaacs, Gertrude. "The Frontier Nursing Service: Family Nursing in Rural Areas." *Clinical Obstetrics and Gynecology* (June 1972), vol. 15.

Mattson, Dale E.; *et al.* "Evaluation of a Program Designed to Produce Rural Physicians." *Journal of Medical Education* (April 1973), vol. 48.

"Nurses: Where Doctors Don't Reach." *Time* (July 22, 1966), vol. 88.

Phillips, Theodore J., D.M.; and Swanson, August G., M.D. "Teaching Family Medicine in Rural Clinical Clerkships: A WAMI Progress Report." *Journal of the American Medical Association* (June 10, 1974).

"Rural Duties Satisfy This Medic." Salt Lake *Tribune*, October 7, 1974.

Schwarz, M. Roy, M.D. "WAMI – An Experiment in Regional Medical Education." *Western Journal of Medicine* (October 1974), vol. 121, no. 4.

Silver, Henry K.; *et al.* "The Pediatric Nurse Practitioner Program." *Journal of the American Medical Association* (April 22, 1968), vol. 204, no. 4.

Sorenson, Jerold G. "An Independent Practice Association HMO: It Works in Grand Junction, Colorado." Salt Lake City, 1975. Unpublished manuscript written for the Intermountain Regional Medical Program.

Stehr, D. E., M.D. "Description of the Illinois Medical Student Loan Fund Program." Bloomington, Illinois. April 1972.

U.S. Department of Agriculture, Rural Development Service. *Health Services in Rural America.* Agriculture Information Bulletin No. 362. Washington, D.C.: U.S. Department of Agriculture. July 1973.

U.S. Department of Health, Education, and Welfare. *National Health Service Corps.* Washington, D.C.: U.S. Government Printing Office.

University of Utah, Department of Family and Community Medicine. *Utah Medex Project Handbook.* Salt Lake City: University of Utah.

10

A Final Word

The models in chapter 9 are presented as being representative of successful rural health care efforts throughout the nation and because they are rather advanced in nature. But by no means can they be considered an all-inclusive picture of current rural health activities.

Aside from other projects not discussed in this book, there are also the support activities of many people and groups that are extremely important to improved rural health. Medical schools, for example, have been involved in getting better health care to rural residents since the problem came into national prominence in the late 1940s. These schools are still looking for new ways in which to provide their rural inhabitants with better health care.

The University of Utah College of Medicine has developed a physician placement program, according to Robert Anderson,[1] administrator with the Department of Family and Community Medicine's Physician Shortage project. This program recruits and places physicians in rural Utah areas and then attempts to retrain them by such methods as its Rural Outreach Physician Education (ROPE) program.

[1]Personal interview, June 16, 1975.

The program contacts physicians felt to be teetering on the brink of leaving their rural practices, and each is invited to come to the university's medical center for a "tailor-made" course designed for his or her individual needs. As of this writing, twelve physicians participated in the ROPE program last year, and thirty more are waiting to take part. Course length is flexible, with most physicians studying for as long as three months or as short as three weeks. The medical school provides a *locum tenum* to cover the practices of physicians participating in the ROPE program; and, while a fee is charged for that, there is no fee for the continuing education.

A second major program is a satellite of the Utah school's Family Practice Department, opened July 1, 1975, in Vernal, Utah. Three full-time faculty members, plus a total interdisciplinary team of midwives, pharmacists, psychologists, Medexes, and nurses provides health care to Vernal area residents. Family practice residents are rotated in and out of the satellite clinic.

The Utah Rural Health Program is also establishing small health care systems in the communities of Panguitch, Escalante, Circleville, Fillmore, Delta, and Duchesne.

At the University of Colorado Medical Center in Denver, the main rural health program is the Student Health Program for Migrant Farmworkers and Rural Poor, devised by the Departments of Pediatrics and Preventive Medicine. Funded by the Colorado-Wyoming Regional Medical Program, it began in 1970.

Senior medical and dental students plus student nurses are divided into teams representing each profession and sent to areas throughout the state where farmworkers gather, with the bulk of the work being done at eighteen Head Start and day care centers, says Dr. Stephen Barnett,[2] project director. Here, students do pre-screening such as audio and visual tests. Later a faculty doctor performs the physical examination; data from the two procedures are pooled and reviewed and a plan of action is established for each problem.

Clinics, set up for the adult population, are held almost anywhere – in mobile vans, a practitioner's office, or perhaps in a vacant building in the farm camp. Home visits are an important part of the student's role, especially where follow-up care is concerned.

---

[2]Telephone interview, June 9, 1975.

Nevada's two-year School of Medical Sciences in Reno attempts to provide additional rural health care through its Rural Family Health Maintenance Program. According to John Moss,[3] who is in charge of program development, first- and second-year medical students go into the rural areas with a team of health professionals and a faculty physician or a doctor from the area. These students perform complete physicals, plus lab work and follow-up. Sixteen teams go out two weekends each year, providing 32 weekends of care for people in isolated rural areas.

Medical Societies, Committees, and Rural Health

Another group frequently active in rural health problems is the state medical society which often establishes a rural health committee, a trend that began when the National Council on Rural Health was formed in 1945. Currently, however, three of the Intermountain Area states have no state medical society rural health committees; two of those, Idaho and Montana, have no state medical society-sponsored programs that aim at only their rural regions, according to spokesmen at the state medical societies.

Nevada is the other state without a rural health committee. However, Nevada does have a Governor's Rural Health Action Committee, established in January 1974 at a meeting of the Nevada Rural Health Conference held at the University of Nevada in Reno. It is funded by the Mountain States Regional Medical Program and consists of fifteen to twenty people from all phases of rural health care life – consumers, educators, doctors, nurses, directors of welfare (to name a few). There are five subcommittees under this main organization.

This past year, the committee came up with three bills that went to the state legislature, according to Melba Holderman,[4] chairwoman. One was for the revocation of the basic science law, which required all physicians entering into a practice in the state to be tested on their knowledge of basic science, and might have deterred older physicians from semiretiring in Nevada. This went into effect July 1, 1975.

Another bill to increase funding to the Nevada State Division of Health, so that the two more public health nurses could be hired

[3]Telephone interview, June 13, 1975.

[4]Telephone interview, April 18, 1975.

to serve outlying areas, was tabled, and a third, whose purpose was to provide Nevada with a state health educator, failed.

The Governor's Rural Health Action Committee has been active in working with state legislators concerning an Emergency Medical Services program in Nevada and, at present, is endorsing the use of fully trained ambulance drivers, stating that all applicants must have eighty hours of training to qualify for the job. The committee has also requested that laws licensing school bus drivers be changed so that all must have first aid training. This request was granted.

The Wyoming State Medical Society sponsors two scientific programs for physicians each year, to help them keep current on innovations in medicine, says Robert Smith,[5] executive secretary. The society has also been involved in outreach programs where it assists in the placement of physician extenders throughout the state and provides a monthly recruitment bulletin to communities seeking physicians so these communities know that there are doctors interested in coming to Wyoming.

Says Smith, "We find out about interested physicians through the AMA placement service, by personal reference, or through those who write and inquire. We send these people information on Wyoming and let them know a little bit about the economic status and so on of the towns that are interested in physicians. Then we get in touch with the communities and encourage them not only to write to the physician but to call him and arrange for a visit."

Utah's Committee on Rural Health, says its chairman, Dr. Keith Hooker,[6] chief of the emergency room at Utah Valley Hospital in Provo, tries to work at the grass roots level. The committee would like to see more rural young men and women with spouses who also have rural backgrounds enter into medical school. Currently, the committee is looking for someone to represent rural interests in the state and be on the University of Utah's Medical Admissions Committee. The committee, says Hooker, is also a liaison for people seeking a rural practice.

"The main purpose of the rural health committee in Colorado," says Dr. S. Jack Locke of Lamar,[7] chairman of the Colorado Committee on Rural Health, "is to educate the physicians and the

[5]Telephone interview, March 11, 1975.

[6]Telephone interview, May 20, 1975, and speech, May 21, 1975.

[7]Telephone interview, June 4, 1975.

public as to what can be done about rural health. We try to involve and interest the rural communities and the state and stress to them that they can solve their own medical problems if they so choose."

The committee, which meets once a month, was planning what Locke called a "humdinger" statewide rural health conference in October 1975 at Colorado State University in Ft. Collins. "We're going to involve twenty or so different types of people; everyone involved in health care delivery that we can get our hands on — doctors, pharmacists, county commissioners, dentists, health planners, lab technicians, hospital administrators, nurses, physician assistants — the whole picture."

His committee has looked at most rural health projects being tried across the nation today; he feels that by including a variety of people involved in health care, a different approach is being used, and he hopes participants leave the state conference thinking "we should have been doing this years ago." Many of the committee's ideas do not explicitly include doctors, and Locke believes that this will not only involve others with the problems and solutions of rural health care, but also intensify the need for full medical leadership by the M.D.s.

One of the committee's goals is to develop more interest in preceptorship programs across the state, both among the state's medical college and eight nursing schools and among the physicians. The rural health committee also hopes to establish some sort of program in which specialists will travel to rural communities on a regular basis. To do this, says Locke, "You have to say, 'Look, you're a doctor and you're not as busy as you could be and you live in Denver. What is your responsibility to rural health?' The conventional ones say that the people must come into the city to see them, but the less conventional doctors see the validity of the concept, and they go one day a month to, say, Vernal, Utah. Then twenty families won't have to go to Salt Lake City, money is kept in the community, and care is given to the people who wouldn't go into Salt Lake for treatment."

Not the Last Word

The rural health activities briefly discussed are not the last word in rural health care, nor are they meant to be. Instead, it is hoped that this presentation will be a basis for continued work and study and will stimulate additional efforts to improve the Intermountain Region's rural health – efforts that will result in residents having access to good health care and who can therefore enjoy a better quality of living.

Index